Surgical Oncology in the Community Cancer Center

Guest Editor

FREDERICK L. GREENE, MD

SURGICAL ONCOLOGY CLINICS OF NORTH AMERICA

www.surgonc.theclinics.com

Consulting Editor
NICHOLAS J. PETRELLI, MD

July 2011 • Volume 20 • Number 3

SAUNDERS an imprint of ELSEVIER, Inc.

W.B. SAUNDERS COMPANY
A Division of Elsevier Inc.

1600 John F. Kennedy Boulevard • Suite 1800 • Philadelphia, PA 19103-2899

http://www.theclinics.com

SURGICAL ONCOLOGY CLINICS OF NORTH AMERICA Volume 20, Number 3
July 2011 ISSN 1055-3207, ISBN-13: 978-1-4557-0803-1

Editor: Jessica Demetriou

Surgical Oncology Clinics of North America (ISSN 1055-3207) is published quarterly by Elsevier Inc., 360 Park Avenue South, New York, NY 10010-1710. Months of publication are January, April, July, and October. Business and Editorial Offices: 1600 John F. Kennedy Blvd., Ste. 1800, Philadelphia, PA 19103-2899. Customer Service Office: 3251 Riverport Lane, Maryland Heights, MO 63043. Periodicals postage paid at New York, NY and additional mailing offices. Subscription prices are $241.00 per year (US individuals), $357.00 (US institutions) $119.00 (US student/resident), $277.00 (Canadian individuals), $444.00 (Canadian institutions), $171.00 (Canadian student/resident), $346.00 (foreign individuals), $444.00 (foreign institutions), and $171.00 (foreign student/resident). Foreign air speed delivery is included in all *Clinics* subscription prices. All prices are subject to change without notice. **POSTMASTER**: Send address changes to *Surgical Oncology Clinics of North America*, Elsevier Health Science Division, Subscription Customer Service, 3251 Riverport Lane, Maryland Heights, MO 63043. **Customer Service: 1-800-654-2452 (US and Canada). 314-447-8871 (outside U.S. and Canada). Fax: 314-447-8029.** E-mail: journalscustomerservice-usa@elsevier.com (for print support); **journalsonline support-usa@elsevier.com** (for online support).

Reprints. For copies of 100 or more, of articles in this publication, please contact the Commercial Reprints Department, Elsevier Inc., 360 Park Avenue South, New York, New York 10010-1710. Tel. 212-633-3813; Fax: 212-462-1935; E-mail: reprints@elsevier.com.

Surgical Oncology Clinics of North America is covered in *MEDLINE/PubMed (Index Medicus)* and *EMBASE/ Excerpta Medica, Current Contents/Clinical Medicine,* and *ISI/BIOMED*.

Printed and bound by CPI Group (UK) Ltd, Croydon, CR0 4YY
Transferred to Digital Print 2011

Contributors

CONSULTING EDITOR

NICHOLAS J. PETRELLI, MD
Bank of America Endowed Medical Director, Helen F. Graham Cancer Center at
Christiana Care Health System, Newark, Delaware; Professor of Surgery, Thomas
Jefferson University, Philadelphia, Pennsylvania

GUEST EDITOR

FREDERICK L. GREENE, MD
Chairman and Surgical Residency Program Director, Department of Surgery, Carolinas
Medical Center, Charlotte, North Carolina

AUTHORS

KATHLEEN G. ALLEN, MD
Surgical Oncologist, Comprehensive Breast Care Center of Tampa Bay, Morton Plant
Hospital, Clearwater, Florida

ASIM AMIN, MD, PhD
Department of Medicine, Carolinas Medical Center, Blumenthal Cancer Center,
Charlotte, North Carolina

LISA BAILEY, MD, FACS
Bay Area Breast Surgeons, Inc, Oakland, California

LOUIS H. BARR, MD, FACS
Medical Director, Florida Hospital Cancer Institute, Orlando, Florida

AARON D. BLEZNAK, MD, FACS
Vice Chair, Operations and Clinical Affairs; Assistant Medical Director, LVPG Surgery,
Department of Surgery, Lehigh Valley Health Network, John and Dorothy Morgan
Cancer Center, Allentown, Pennsylvania; Assistant Professor of Surgery, University
of South Florida School of Medicine, Tampa, Florida

LISA E. BLUMENCRANZ, BA
Research Assistant, Comprehensive Breast Care Center of Tampa Bay, Morton Plant
Hospital, Clearwater, Florida

PETER W. BLUMENCRANZ, MD
Medical Director, Comprehensive Breast Care Center of Tampa Bay, Morton Plant
Hospital, Clearwater, Florida

JANE CROFTON, RN, BSN, OCN, CCRP
Administrative Director, Oncology Research and Cancer Registry, Florida Hospital Cancer
Institute, Orlando, Florida

ANTHONY P. D'ANDREA, MS
Medical Research Assistant, Division of Colorectal Surgery, Marks Colorectal Surgical Foundation, Lankenau Hospital, Wynnewood, Pennsylvania

DIANA DICKSON-WITMER, MD, FACS
Associate Medical Director, Department of Surgery, Helen F. Graham Cancer Center at Christiana Care Health System, Newark, Delaware; Assistant Clinical Professor of Surgery, Thomas Jefferson Medical College, Philadelphia, Pennsylvania

MARTIN FEUERMAN, MS
Health Outcomes Research-Biostatistics, Winthrop-University Hospital, Mineola, New York

JOSEPH L. FRENKEL, MD
Minimally Invasive Colorectal Surgery and Rectal Cancer Fellow, Division of Colorectal Surgery, Lankenau Hospital, Wynnewood, Pennsylvania

JULES E. GARBUS, MD
Clinical Assistant Professor of Surgery, State University of New York at Stony Brook, New York, New York

FREDERICK L. GREENE, MD
Chairman and Surgical Residency Program Director, Department of Surgery, Carolinas Medical Center, Charlotte, North Carolina

CHISTOPHER E. GREENLEAF, MD
General Surgery Resident, Division of Graduate Medical Education, Lankenau Hospital, Wynnewood, Pennsylvania

ERIN M. HANNA, MD
General Surgery Resident, Department of General Surgery, Carolinas Medical Center, Charlotte, North Carolina

DAVID A. IANNITTI, MD, FACS
Hepato-Pancreato-Biliary Surgery, Department of General Surgery, Carolinas Medical Center, Charlotte, North Carolina

J. BENJAMIN JACKSON III, MD
PGY-4, Department of Orthopaedic Surgery, Carolinas Medical Center, Charlotte, North Carolina

JOHN S. KENNEDY, MD, FACS
DeKalb Surgical Associates, DeKalb Medical Center, Decatur, Georgia

JEFFREY S. KNEISL, MD, FACS
Medical Director, Blumenthal Cancer Center, Charlotte, North Carolina

ALISON L. LAIDLEY, MD, FACS, FRCS(C)
Texas Breast Specialists, Dallas, Texas

KWAN N. LAU, MD
Hepato-Pancreato-Biliary Surgery, Department of General Surgery, Carolinas Medical Center, Charlotte, North Carolina

A. MARILYN LEITCH, MD, FACS
Professor of Surgery, University of Texas Medical Center, Dallas, Texas

YU-HSIN ANNIE LIN, MD
Resident, Surgery Residency Program, Florida Hospital, Orlando, Florida

JOHN H. MARKS, MD
Medical Director, Lankenau Hospital Colorectal Center; Chief of Colorectal Surgery, Main Line Health Systems; Director of Minimally Invasive Colorectal Surgery and Rectal Cancer Management Fellowship, Division of Colorectal Surgery, Lankenau Hospital; Professor, Lankenau Institute of Medical Research, Wynnewood, Pennsylvania

JOHN B. MARTINIE, MD
Hepato-Pancreato-Biliary Surgery, Department of General Surgery, Carolinas Medical Center, Charlotte, North Carolina

MARSHA CRISCIO NELSON, MD, MPH
Department of Surgery, Carolinas Medical Center, Charlotte, North Carolina

H. JAMES NORTON, PhD
Director, Department of Biostatistics, Carolinas Medical Center, Charlotte, North Carolina

DAVID M. OTA, MD, FACS
ACOSOG Group Co-Chair, Department of Surgery, Duke University, Durham, North Carolina

BRYAN E. PALIS, MA
Quality Improvement Information Analyst, American College of Surgeons, Commission on Cancer, National Cancer Data Base, Chicago, Illinois

DEAN P. PAPPAS, MD
Clinical Assistant Professor of Surgery, State University of New York at Stony Brook, New York, New York

EMILY J. PENMAN, MD, FACS
Medical Director, Department of Surgery, Helen F. Graham Cancer Center at Christiana Care Health System, Newark, Delaware; Associate Professor of Surgery, Thomas Jefferson Medical College, Philadelphia, Pennsylvania

MAURA PIERETTI, PhD
Scientific Director, Molecular Diagnostic Laboratory, BayCare Laboratory, BayCare Health System, Clearwater, Florida

MARK K. REAMES, MD
Attending Surgeon, Sanger Heart and Vascular Institute, Charlotte, North Carolina

WILLIAM P. REED, MD
Professor of Surgery, State University of New York at Stony Brook, New York; Chair, Department of Surgery, Winthrop-University Hospital, Mineola, New York

JONATHAN C. SALO, MD
Attending Surgeon, Division of Surgical Oncology, Department of General Surgery, Carolinas Medical Center, Blumenthal Cancer Center, Charlotte, North Carolina

DAVID SINDRAM, MD, PhD
Hepato-Pancreato-Biliary Surgery, Department of General Surgery, Carolinas Medical Center, Charlotte, North Carolina

ANDREW K. STEWART, MA
Manager, National Cancer Data Base, American College of Surgeons, Commission on Cancer, Chicago, Illinois

RYAN Z. SWAN, MD
Hepato-Pancreato-Biliary Surgery, Department of General Surgery, Carolinas Medical Center, Charlotte, North Carolina

GARY UNZEITIG, MD, FACS
Attending Surgeon, Doctors Hospital of Laredo, Laredo, Texas

RICHARD L. WHITE Jr, MD, FACS
Co-Director of Immunotherapy; Chief, Division of Surgical Oncology, Carolinas Medical Center, Blumenthal Cancer Center, Charlotte, North Carolina

DAVID P. WINCHESTER, MD, FACS
Clinical Professor of Surgery, University of Chicago Pritzker School of Medicine, Evanston Hospital, Evanston; Medical Director, Cancer Programs, American College of Surgeons, Chicago, Illinois

Contents

care navigators is also discussed. Strong hospital administrative support and clinical research staff are crucial for success.

Primary liver tumors are a common clinical problem in the United States and worldwide. Resection has historically been used to treat liver lesions. Commonly used liver-directed therapies include transarterial chemoembolization, selective internal radiation therapy, and ablative therapy. Only ablative therapy can cause direct destruction of the targeted tissue. The commercially available modalities in the United States are all based on thermoablative technology. This article examines the various ablative technologies and their application, as well as how these procedures can be performed safely and with optimal outcomes, in a community cancer center.

Lymphatic mapping and sentinel lymph node (SLN) biopsy have become the standard of care for staging the axilla in patients with invasive breast cancer. Current histologic methods for SLN evaluation have limitations, including subjectivity, limited sensitivity, and lack of standardization. The discovery of molecular markers to detect metastases has been reported over the last 2 decades. The authors review the historical development of these markers and the clinical use of one of the molecular platforms in 478 patients at their institution. Controversies and future directions are discussed.

Pancreatic resection can be performed safely in the community-based hospital setting only when appropriate systems are in place for patient selection and preoperative, operative, and postoperative care. Pancreatic surgery cannot be performed optimally without considerable investment in, and coordination of, multiple departments. Delivery of high-quality pancreatic cancer care demands a rigorous assessment of the hospital structure and the processes through which this care is delivered; however, when a hospital makes the considerable effort to establish the necessary systems required for delivery of quality pancreatic cancer care, the community and hospital will benefit substantially.

Rectal cancer management benefits from a multidisciplinary approach involving medical and radiation oncology as well as surgery. Presented are the current dominant issues in rectal cancer management with an emphasis on our treatment algorithm at the Lankenau Medical Center. By basing surgical decisions on the downstaged rectal cancer we explore how sphincter preservation can be extended even for cancers of the distal 3 cm of the rectum. TATA and TEM techniques can be used to effectively treat cancer from an oncologic standpoint while maintaining a high quality of life through sphincter preservation and avoidance of a permanent colostomy. We review the results of our efforts, including the use of advanced laparoscopy in the surgical management of low rectal cancers.

We report our initial experience with minimally-invasive esophagectomy in 32 patients at Carolinas Medical Center, a community academic medical center. Indications for surgery were adenocarcinoma in 27, squamous cell carcinoma in 3, and benign stricture in 2. Transthoracic Ivor-Lewis esophagectomy with laparoscopy and thoracoscopy was performed in 28, a 3-stage esophagectomy in 3, and transhaital esophagectomy in 1. There was no operative mortality and median hospital stay was 10.5 days for patients treated with minimally invasive esophagectomy. This compares with an operative mortality of 8.9% and median hospital stay of 17 days for open esophagectomy in our institution.

Immune-based therapies for cancer are now commonplace. Cytokine therapy, including interferon and interleukin-2, is safe in the community setting. The US Food and Drug Administration has recently approved sipuleucel-T for the treatment of advanced prostate cancer, the first therapeutic cancer vaccine to meet this level of efficacy. The therapeutic use of monoclonal antibodies directed against proteins controlling various cell functions, including growth and modulation of immune response, has become so pervasive that the oncologist, whether surgeon or medical oncologist, must be familiar with indications, contraindications, and the associated toxicities.

In the USA, 80% of patients with breast cancer are treated by community breast surgeons. NCDB data indicate that there are only small differences in outcomes between lower volume cancer programs and higher volume programs. There is some evidence that breast cancer patients of high-volume breast focused surgeons may have improved outcomes. This article discusses the challenges community breast surgeons face and some ways that the quality of care could be monitored and improved. Quality reporting programs of the Commission on Cancer and Mastery of Breast Surgery Program of the American Society of Breast Surgeons are recommended as tools to track and improve outcomes in breast cancer care.

The breast center concept developed in response to a fragmented inefficient system to evaluate and manage patients with diseases of the breast. The National Accreditation Program for Breast Centers (NAPBC) accreditation is granted only to those centers that have voluntarily committed to provide the best in the diagnosis and treatment of breast cancer and are able to comply with the established NAPBC standards. Each center must undergo a rigorous evaluation and review of its performance and compliance with the NAPBC standards. The NAPBC is in the process of defining the most efficient methods of data collection for the NAPBC-accredited programs.

The National Cancer Data Base (NCDB) provides feedback on adherence to National Quality Forum (NQF)–endorsed measures to promote best outcomes in colorectal cancer. We examined the care delivered to patients with colorectal cancer at our institution and developed a protocol to enhance nodal retrieval and to ensure that patients with fewer than 12 nodes are considered for adjuvant chemotherapy. Few patients met the NQF criteria for adjuvant radiation. A protocol was developed to address this issue, and this provides a model for use in a multidisciplinary effort to improve adherence to measures associated with best outcomes in colorectal cancer.

RELATED INTEREST

Surgical Clinics of North America, April 2011 (Vol. 91, Issue 2)
Update on Surgical Palliative Care
Geoffrey P. Dunn, MD, FACS, *Guest Editor*
Available at: http://www.surgical.theclinics.com/

VISIT THE CLINICS ONLINE!

Access your subscription at:
www.theclinics.com

Foreword

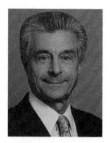

Nicholas J. Petrelli, MD
Consulting Editor

The guest editor for this issue of the *Surgical Oncology Clinics of North America* is Frederick L. Greene, MD. Dr Greene is Chairman and Director of Surgical Education at the Carolinas Medical Center. Dr Greene is also Clinical Professor in the Department of Surgery at the University of North Carolina at Chapel Hill. He has held this position since 1997.

This is a unique issue of the *Surgical Oncology Clinics of North America* since it deals with the subject matter of surgical oncology in the community cancer center. It is important to note that 85% of cancer patients in the United States are diagnosed at hospitals in their communities. The remaining 15% are diagnosed at National Cancer Institute (NCI)-designated cancer centers, which are academic institutions in mainly urban areas. Many patients are not treated at the NCI-designated cancer centers because of distance from home, personal, or economic reasons. However, as noted in this issue of the *Surgical Oncology Clinics of North America*, cancer care in many community cancer centers can be delivered with high quality and excellent outcomes. Some community cancer centers, such as our own at the Helen F. Graham Cancer Center, have even established successful programs of translational cancer research.

Although not discussed in this issue, in 2007 the NCI launched the Community Cancer Centers Program (NCCCP) to evaluate the best methods to enhance access to care, especially for those individuals with health care disparities and, at the same time, expanding research within a community setting. I hope to have the NCCCP be a topic for a future issue of the *Surgical Oncology Clinics of North America*.

Surg Oncol Clin N Am 20 (2011) xiii–xiv
doi:10.1016/j.soc.2011.02.001
1055-3207/11/$ – see front matter © 2011 Elsevier Inc. All rights reserved.

surgonc.theclinics.com

I'd like to thank Dr Greene and the authors for this unique issue of the *Surgical Oncology Clinics of North America*. It demonstrates the excellent care that patients can receive in community cancer centers.

Nicholas J. Petrelli, MD
Helen F. Graham Cancer Center
4701 Ogletown-Stanton Road, Suite 1213
Newark, DE 19713, USA

E-mail address:
npetrelli@christianacare.org

Preface

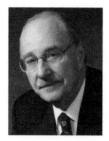

Frederick L. Greene, MD
Guest Editor

It has been an honor for me to serve as guest editor for this issue of *Surgical Oncology Clinics of North America* dedicated to surgical oncology in the community cancer center. There is no question that outstanding surgical oncologic care is the mainstay for the majority of people having cancer in the United States. Dr Nicholas Petrelli, consulting editor of *Surgical Oncology Clinics of North America* and Director of the Helen F. Graham Cancer Center at Christiana Care Health System in Delaware, has a keen interest in this concept and I appreciate the choice of this topic for publication.

I have had the great pleasure of working with the Commission on Cancer of the American College of Surgeons for a number of years and, as a hospital surveyor, I continue to be impressed and proud of the excellent oncology care given by our community hospitals throughout the United States. While surgical management of cancer patients has been intertwined with medical oncology and radiation oncology care over the last several decades, the role of the surgeon in the primary management of cancer continues to be of great importance.

In this issue of *Surgical Oncology Clinics of North America* several specific cancer issues are highlighted as evidenced by reports of excellence in rectal cancer care using new surgical concepts authored by John Marks and his colleagues at the Lankenau Hospital in Wynnewood, Pennsylvania. Ablative techniques for both primary and metastatic liver tumors are reported by David Iannitti and his colleagues at the Carolinas Medical Center in Charlotte. Management of breast cancer with modern sentinel node technology is reported by Peter Blumencranz from Clearwater, FL. In addition to these specific areas, Dr Jonathan Salo outlines the approach to minimal access surgical management of patients with esophageal cancer and Richard White and Asim Amin describe their approach to immunotherapy of solid tumors and the introduction of these concepts into the community setting.

One of our great challenges is to increase the accrual of patients to clinical trials and to utilize the great resources that community cancer centers bring to the science of cancer treatment. David Ota, the co-chair of the American College of Surgeons Oncology Group (ACOSOG), and his colleagues describe the opportunities for entering patients into clinical trials by community surgeons and other physicians dedicated to cancer care. These concepts are also highlighted in the overview offered by Diana

Surg Oncol Clin N Am 20 (2011) xv–xvi
doi:10.1016/j.soc.2011.01.012
surgonc.theclinics.com

Dickson-Witmer as she and her colleagues describe the challenges for breast cancer care in a community setting. Dr David P. Winchester, who has been a remarkable thought leader not only in breast cancer management but also as medical director of the Commission on Cancer, has spearheaded the effort for accreditation of breast cancer care in the community setting. His description of the National Accreditation Program for Breast Centers (NAPBC) is an important step in increasing modern breast cancer care through the utilization of quality indicators. The importance of the cancer registry is highlighted in Marsha Nelson's report assessing the rate of lumpectomy versus mastectomy procedures in the community setting and debating whether particular forms of cancer care should be considered as quality benchmarks. Other outstanding contributions round out the important issues and are listed in the table of contents.

One definition of "community" is a group of people having common interests. There is no doubt that the articles contained in this issue of *Surgical Oncology Clinics of North America* offer a microcosm of the excellent work that can be done and should be done in surgical management of cancer patients at the community cancer center. The benchmark of future care will be multidisciplinary decision-making prior to any treatment.

I wish to thank all of the authors who submitted manuscripts for this issue and who have taken the time from their busy schedules to prepare these reports. In addition I would like to thank Catherine Bewick and Jessica Demetriou, representing Elsevier Health Sciences, who have given me outstanding support in the development of this issue. Finally I wish to recognize all of the outstanding surgical specialists who give their time and intellect in the management of our cancer patients. I anticipate that the concepts reviewed in this issue will be examples of the exciting and important advances in cancer management that will characterize community care in the future.

Frederick L. Greene, MD
Department of Surgery
Carolinas Medical Center
1000 Blythe Boulevard, MEB 601
Charlotte, NC 28203, USA

E-mail address:
Frederick.Greene@carolinashealthcare.org

Building a Community-Based Cancer Center Program

Jeffrey S. Kneisl, MD[a],*,[1], J. Benjamin Jackson III, MD[b]

KEYWORDS
- Cancer program • Commission on cancer • Quality

The development of a successful cancer center program is not limited to an academic environment; in fact, more than 85% of patients in the United States will receive their initial diagnosis or care at a community cancer center.[1,2] The creation and improvement of community cancer programs is critical to the advancement of cancer care in this country.[3] Among their many functions, cancer centers promote excellence in cancer care in the community, apply national normative standards of care, optimize the delivery of care, improve access to clinical trials, and measure and report cancer metrics to entities such as the National Cancer Database.[4]

Historically, formal processes for continuously understanding, managing, and controlling cancer have been driven by surgeons through the mechanisms of the American College of Surgeon's (ACS) Commission on Cancer (CoC). Established in 1922, the ACS CoC was formed as a consortium of professional organizations dedicated to improving survival and quality of life for patients with cancer through standard-setting, prevention, research, education, and monitoring of comprehensive quality of care.

Standards for the evaluation of cancer clinics and registries were first published in 1930 by the ACS Committee on the Treatment of Malignant Disease. The first surveys of cancer clinics were conducted in 1931. Continuously revised and expanded, these

The authors have nothing to disclose.

[a] Department of Orthopaedic Surgery, Blumenthal Cancer Center, 1025 Morehead Medical Drive, Suite 300, Charlotte, NC 28204, USA

[b] PGY-4, Department of Orthopaedic Surgery, Carolinas Medical Center, 1025 Morehead Medical Drive, Suite 300, Charlotte, NC 28204, USA

[1] Author's Note: Dr Jeffrey Kneisl has been the Chairman of the Carolinas Medical Center Cancer Committee since 1995, and has been the Medical Director of the Blumenthal Cancer Center since 1999. He is a practicing orthopaedic oncologist.

* Corresponding author. Department of Orthopaedic Surgery, 1025 Morehead Medical Drive, Suite 300, Charlotte, NC 28204.

E-mail address: jeffrey.kneisl@carolinashealthcare.org

doi:10.1016/j.soc.2011.03.001
1055-3207/11/$ – see front matter © 2011 Elsevier Inc. All rights reserved.
surgonc.theclinics.com

standards define the development process for a cancer program. The most recent standards were published in 2009.[5]

This introductory article provides a primer for understanding the mechanism for building a community-based cancer program. The pillars of this process include understanding established standards and guidelines of the CoC, the different community cancer program categories, the accreditation process, the role of physician leadership, and the need for institutional support. The seven CoC cancer programs applicable to the community setting and the requirements for accreditation in each are explored. For a more thorough and complete description, the reader is directed to the ACS CoC guidelines.

CANCER CENTER VERSUS CANCER PROGRAM

Large academic cancer centers have no monopoly on the treatment of cancer. For instance, although the NCI Cancer Center Programs make significant contributions in cancer research that are key to understanding, preventing, and treating this disease, only 15% of patients in the United States are diagnosed and receive their initial treatment at NCI-designated cancer centers. Thus, 85% of cancer care is provided in the community setting. According to CoC statistics for 2010, 71% of cancer care is provided in one of the 1400 CoC accredited programs.

The term *cancer center* is neither codified nor copyrighted. According to Simone,[2] a cancer center is best described as "a formal organization of diverse and complimentary specialists who work on the cancer problem together and simultaneously rather than serially. The center is under sufficient central authority to focus efforts and organize resources for the efficient and synergistic accomplishments of its goals in patient care and/or research." This term suggests a physical proximity of services that complements the efficient and reproducible delivery of care.

A cancer program extends the cancer center concept dramatically. A cancer program not only addresses the significant and immediate needs of diagnosis and treatment but also provides community screening, long-term follow-up with data registry reporting, and posttreatment surveillance. In addition to meeting the needs of the patient, a cancer program provides cancer education to the community and disease-specific certification to the medical staff.

THE ACCREDITATIONS PROGRAM

Through the CoC Accreditations Program, any hospital or treatment center that seeks to improve the quality of care within its community can voluntarily commit to comply with CoC standards designed for facilities of similar size. After conforming to the guidelines (discussed later) a program can then apply for accreditation. Accreditation is granted only to facilities that have undergone a thorough and rigorous evaluation and performance review for compliance with the CoC standards. To maintain accreditation, facilities with accredited cancer programs must undergo an on-site review every 3 years.

All hospitals and freestanding treatment facilities are eligible to participate in the CoC Accreditation Program. The five elements key to the success of a CoC Accredited Cancer Program are (1) clinical services, (2) cancer committee/leadership body, (3) cancer conferences, (4) quality improvement program, and (5) cancer registry and database. By design, compliance with the CoC standards established for any one of the CoC-defined cancer program categories (**Table 1**) promotes improved patient care.

COC CANCER PROGRAM CATEGORIES

For the purposes of this introductory article, those seeking to build a community level cancer program will most likely be targeting accreditation at a Community Hospital Comprehensive Cancer Program (COMP) level or lower designation (**Table 2**). A COMP is defined by the CoC as a facility that accessions 650 or more newly diagnosed cancer cases each year and provides a full range of diagnostic and treatment services that are available on site or by referral. The members of the medical staff are board certified in the major medical specialties, including oncology, where applicable. This community-based program is the only that requires participation in clinical research. Participation when training resident physicians is optional.

A Community Hospital Cancer Program (CHCP) is defined by the CoC as a facility that accessions between 100 and 649 newly diagnosed cancer cases each year and provides a full range of diagnostic and treatment services, but referral for a portion of treatment is common. The members of the medical staff are board certified in the major medical specialties. Facilities may participate in clinical research. Participation in the training of resident physicians is optional. Requirements of COMPs and CHCPs are provided in **Box 1**.

Fundamentally, the following four programs are required to provide the same basic services, despite having programs that accrue fewer than 100 newly diagnosed cancer cases per year. It is possible, and most likely, that many requirements are met through referring services to or coordinating services with other facilities or local agencies.

The Hospital Associate Cancer Program is defined by the CoC as a facility that accrues between 50 and 99 newly diagnosed cancer cases each year and has a limited range of diagnostic and treatment services on site. Other services are available by referral. Clinical research is not required. Participation in the training of resident physicians is optional.

The Affiliate Hospital Cancer Program is defined by the CoC as a facility that accrues fewer than 50 newly diagnosed cancer cases each year, has limited access to services on site, and forms a partnership with a CoC-accredited sponsoring hospital to provide access to the full range of diagnostic and treatment services. Clinical research is not required. Participation in the training of resident physicians is optional.

The Integrated Cancer Program offers one treatment modality and forms a partnership with a CoC-accredited hospital to provide access to the full range of diagnostic and treatment services. Participation by the integrated facility in clinical research is optional. Participation in the training of resident physicians is optional, and this category has no minimum caseload requirement.

The Freestanding Cancer Center Program offers a minimum of two treatment modalities, and the full range of diagnostic and treatment services are available by referral. Referral to a CoC-accredited program is preferred. Participation in clinical research is optional. Participation in the training of resident physicians is optional, and this category has no minimum caseload requirement.

COMMUNITY-BASED CANCER CENTER CATEGORIES
Leadership

The quality of the leadership defines the success of the program.[6] Fundamentally, physician leadership is the critical success factor in the creation of a community-based cancer program. It is necessary to forge a commitment among involved oncologic physicians from the disciplines of medical oncology and surgery, radiation oncology, pathology, and radiology. It is also necessary to align the paramedical

Table 1
Cancer program categories

Program	Required Category Goals	Required Coordinators	Minimum Number of Newly Diagnosed Cancer Cases	Minimum Required Percentage Accrual to Clinical Trials
Network Cancer Program (NCP)	Clinical Community outreach Programmatic endeavors Quality improvement	Cancer conference Quality of cancer registry data Quality improvement Community outreach	None	8%
NCI-designated Comprehensive Cancer Program (NCIP)	Cancer conference Clinical Quality improvement	None	None	Exempt
Teaching Hospital Cancer Program (THCP)	Clinical Community outreach Programmatic endeavors Quality improvement	Cancer conference Quality of cancer registry data Quality improvement Community outreach	None	4%
Veterans Affairs Cancer Program (VACP)	Clinical Programmatic endeavors Quality improvement	Cancer conference Quality of cancer registry data Quality improvement, For facilities that qualify, ad hoc or Veterans Integrated Service Networks–assigned coordinators are appointed	None	2%
Pediatric Cancer Program (PCP)	Clinical Clinical research Programmatic endeavors Quality improvement	Cancer conference Quality of cancer registry data Quality improvement Child life or long-term follow-up	None	4%

Program	Components	Description	Number	Percentage
Pediatric Component Cancer Program (PCPC)	Clinical Clinical research Programmatic endeavors Quality improvement	Facility coordinators responsible for activities of the pediatric cancer program Pediatric cancer conference Child life or long-term follow-up	50	4%
Community Hospital Comprehensive Cancer Program (COMP)	Clinical Community outreach Programmatic endeavors Quality improvement	Cancer conference, quality of cancer registry data, quality improvement, community outreach	650	2%
Community Hospital Cancer Program (CHCP)	Clinical Community outreach Programmatic endeavors Quality improvement	Cancer conference Quality of cancer registry data Quality improvement Community outreach	100–649	Exempt
Hospital Associate Cancer Program (HACP)	Clinical Community outreach Programmatic endeavors Quality improvement	Cancer conference Quality of cancer registry data Quality improvement Community outreach	50–99	Exempt
Affiliate Hospital Cancer Program (AFCP)	Clinical Community outreach Programmatic endeavors Quality improvement	Cancer conference Quality of cancer registry data Quality improvement Community outreach	Less than 50	Exempt
Integrated Cancer Program (ICP)	Clinical Community outreach Programmatic endeavors Quality improvement	Cancer conference Quality of cancer registry data Quality improvement Community outreach	None	Exempt
Freestanding Cancer Center Program (FCCP)	Clinical Community outreach Programmatic endeavors Quality improvement	Cancer conference Quality of cancer registry data Quality improvement Community outreach	None	Exempt

Table 2
Community level cancer program designations

Program	Required Category Goals	Required Coordinators	Minimum Number of Newly Diagnosed Cancer Cases
Community Hospital Comprehensive Cancer Program (COMP)	Clinical Community outreach Programmatic endeavors Quality improvement	Cancer conference Quality of cancer registry data Quality improvement Community outreach	650[a]
Community Hospital Cancer Program (CHCP)	Clinical Community outreach Programmatic endeavors Quality improvement	Cancer conference Quality of cancer registry data Quality improvement Community outreach	100–649
Hospital Associate Cancer Program (HACP)	Clinical Community outreach Programmatic endeavors Quality improvement	Cancer conference Quality of cancer registry data Quality improvement Community outreach	50–99
Affiliate Hospital Cancer Program (AFCP)	Clinical Community outreach Programmatic endeavors Quality improvement	Cancer conference Quality of cancer registry data Quality improvement Community outreach	Less than 50
Integrated Cancer Program (ICP)	Clinical Community outreach Programmatic endeavors Quality improvement	Cancer conference Quality of cancer registry data Quality improvement Community outreach	None
Freestanding Cancer Center Program (FCCP)	Clinical Community outreach Programmatic endeavors Quality improvement	Cancer conference Quality of cancer registry data Quality improvement Community outreach	None

[a] 2% must be enrolled in clinical trials.

Box 1
Requirements of COMPs and CHCPs

- Prevention and early detection programs
- Diagnostic clinical laboratory and imaging
- Treatment guidelines
- Medical, surgical, and radiation treatment
- Discharge planning
- American Joint Commission on Cancer (AJCC) or other appropriate staging
- Clinical research
- Oncology nursing and nutritional support
- Counseling, pastoral care, patient and family support
- Pain management, hospice

---

personnel from the cancer data registry, medical records, and medical staff office. The recommended internal structure is a medical staff–supported cancer committee, which follows the requirements and recommendations of the desired CoC designation level. The ACS cancer liaison physician supports the CoC mission specifically, and is required in establishing a new program. Although the ACS liaison physician need not be the leader of the cancer program, nor the chairman of the hospital cancer committee, this role is pivotal to the pursuit of the CoC standards and accreditation process.

Cancer Committee

The current CoC guidelines (2009) require that an accredited CoC program must have a cancer committee consisting of personnel from various disciplines given specific responsibility and accountability through institutional by-laws or policies and procedures (**Box 2**). This committee must be responsible for goal-setting, planning, initiating, implementing, evaluating, and improving all cancer-related activities.

Box 2
Members of the CoC cancer committee

Physician

1. Diagnostic radiologist
2. Pathologist
3. General surgeon
4. Medical oncologist
5. Radiation oncologist (if applicable)

Nonphysician

1. Cancer program administrator
2. Oncology nurse
3. Social worker or case manager
4. Certified tumor registrar
5. Performance improvement or quality management professional

---

These committees at community programs are required to meet at least quarterly. During these meetings, the members must establish goals in clinical care, community outreach, quality improvement, and programmatic improvement. The committee must also establish multidisciplinary conferences, determine the number and specialty of the physicians who must attend, and how often the committees meet to prospectively discuss patient care.[7] The committee is responsible for annually monitoring the number of prospective cases presented and ensuring that patient care is properly staged using the AJCC guidelines. Additionally, clinical care discussions at multidisciplinary conferences are to be prospective and reflect the meaningful use and discussion of applicable National Comprehensive Cancer Network (NCCN) guidelines.

An Evolutionary Process

The authors' institution evolved through the various accreditation stages described in this article. The Carolinas Medical center was designated a CHCP in 1989. At that time, the hospital cancer committee consisted of a handful of community medical oncologists and surgeons who were committed to improving the care of patients with cancer through application of the CoC standards program. Over the ensuing 20 years, Carolinas Medical Center has progressively grown from a single-hospital CHCP to a four-hospital CoC Network Cancer Program. The cancer committee, originally a small group of committed individuals, has morphed into a dedicated team of more than 50 individuals, overseeing nearly 4000 new cancer diagnoses in 2009, and has 11 different multidisciplinary tumor site teams and conferences. Carolinas Heath Care System now has 28 additional affiliated hospitals, many of which are small rural hospitals that will be pursuing associate or affiliate status through the processes described.

SUMMARY

Developing a successful cancer center within the community is achievable. This article provides an understanding of the standards and guidelines of the CoC, the different community cancer center program categories, and the accreditation process. The pivotal roles of institutional support and physician leadership in the development of a successful cancer center have been elucidated. The institution must be willing to commit both financially and with facilities as needed. The physician leader must be able to rally support from many specialties and administrators, while always being a strong advocate for improving the quality of cancer care. The development of an accredited community cancer program, at any level, can ensure awareness and compliance with CoC standards and NCCN guidelines. Following these guidelines can be particularly useful for smaller institution and programs that may have quality–volume relationships with certain cancer diagnoses.[3,8,9] With these aspects in place, a successful community cancer program will follow.

REFERENCES

1. NCI Community Cancer Centers Program. Pilot: 2007–2010. Available at: http://www.cancer.gov. Accessed August 15, 2010.
2. Simone JV. Understanding cancer centers. J Clin Oncol 2002;20:4503–7.
3. Neuss MN, Desch CE, McNiff KK, et al. A process of measuring the quality of cancer care: the quality oncology practice initiative. J Clin Oncol 2005;23:6233–9.
4. Hewitt M, Simone JV, editors. Ensuring quality cancer care. Washington, DC: National Academy Press; 1999.

5. American College of Surgeons Commission on Cancer. Cancer program standards. Chicago: American College of Surgeons; 2009.

6. Simone JV. Understanding academic medical centers: Simone's Maxims. Clin Cancer Res 1999;5:2281–5.

7. Greene FL, Gilkerson S, Tedder P, et al. The role of the hospital registry in achieving outcome benchmarks in cancer care. J Surg Oncol 2009;99:497–9.

8. Greene FL. Is volume the most important predictor of outcome in cancer management? J Surg Oncol 2008;97:97–8.

9. Cunningham JD, O'Donnell N, Starker P. Surgical outcomes following pancreatic resection at a low-volume community hospital: do all patients need to be sent to a regional center? Am J Surg 2009;198:227–30.

Breast Conservation Therapy Versus Mastectomy in the Community-Based Setting: Can This Rate Be Used as a Benchmark for Cancer Care?

Marsha Criscio Nelson, MD, MPH[a], H. James Norton, PhD[b], Frederick L. Greene, MD[c],*

KEYWORDS

- Breast carcinoma • Breast conservation • Lumpectomy
- Mastectomy • Treatment • Benchmark

The beginning of the twenty-first century saw the further disappearance of surgical procedures such as the Halsted radical mastectomy, which the newest generation of surgeons will never see, much less perform, except in the occasional rare circumstance. The publication of several prospective, randomized studies demonstrating no difference in survival between mastectomy and breast-conserving surgery, coupled with the paradigm shift to breast carcinoma being considered a systemic disease at the time of diagnosis, led to the promulgation of breast conservation surgery combined with local radiotherapy as a valid treatment modality.[1–3] Low rates of breast conservation therapy (BCT) were initially reported with what seemed to be a slow gain in acceptance of the practice across the United States.[4–7] A multitude of reasons, ranging from surgeon preference to limited access to radiation facilities, were found to influence the choice of surgery in the treatment of early-stage breast cancers.[8,9]

The authors have nothing to disclose.
[a] Department of Surgery, Carolinas Medical Center, 1000 Blythe Boulevard, Charlotte, NC 28203, USA
[b] Department of Biostatistics, Carolinas Medical Center, 1000 Blythe Boulevard, Charlotte, NC 28203, USA
[c] Department of Surgery, Carolinas Medical Center, 1000 Blythe Boulevard, MEB 601, Charlotte, NC 28203, USA
* Corresponding author.
E-mail address: Frederick.Greene@carolinashealthcare.org

Surg Oncol Clin N Am 20 (2011) 427–437
doi:10.1016/j.soc.2011.01.005
1055-3207/11/$ – see front matter © 2011 Elsevier Inc. All rights reserved.

surgonc.theclinics.com

Whereas more recent studies have noted a much higher rate of BCT,[10,11] at least one study found mastectomy rates increasing for women with stage I and stage II cancers.[12]

Regional differences have been detected in the use of BCT since its inception. Studies in the 1990s found that women in the northeast United States had much higher rates of BCT than those in the southeast, southwest, or midwest.[13–15] The south, in particular, has stood out as having one of the lowest rates of BCT.[5] A statewide analysis of North Carolina on the rates of BCT for 6 years found that the rates of BCT range from 7.3% in 1988 to 14.3% in 1993.[16] The reasons cited in the literature for this variation included regional differences in both physician attitudes and patient preferences, as well as older patient age; however, over time, this discrepancy has somewhat diminished.[14]

Most cases of breast cancer in the United States are treated in the community setting. Of the more than 1500 programs accredited by the Commission on Cancer, a consortium established by the American College of Surgeons in 1922 dedicated to improving survival and quality of life for patients with cancer, approximately 70% were community based. The Carolinas Medical Center (CMC), located in Charlotte, North Carolina, is one of the major teaching hospitals in the state with 11 different residency programs and many fellowship training programs. A large academic community hospital and tertiary referral center, CMC treats a large number of patients with breast carcinoma each year. Of the 29,458 new cases of cancer at CMC between 1999 and 2009, breast cancer cases made up almost one-fifth of the total. The authors conducted a retrospective review of the hospital cancer registry to analyze whether mastectomy and BCT rates had changed over the past 11 years at CMC and to determine the factors that may have contributed to this change.

METHODS

The study was conducted at CMC, an 874-bed community hospital. CMC is part of the Carolinas HealthCare System that includes 32 affiliated hospitals in North and South Carolina. The North Carolina Central Cancer Registry collects, processes, and analyzes data on all cancer cases diagnosed among North Carolina residents. Reporting this information is mandatory for all health care providers, although most of the data are furnished by hospitals. The CMC Cancer Registry was established in July 1987 and initially collected data only from the main hospital. The registry obtained network status during the Commission on Cancer accreditation program in 2004 and was expanded to include cancer data from other hospitals in the Carolinas HealthCare System.

The CMC tumor registry was queried to identify patients diagnosed with breast carcinoma from January 1, 1999, through December 31, 2009, who underwent their initial surgical therapy at the main hospital. A sample of approximately one-fourth of the cases identified was reviewed. From this sample, the authors excluded patients who did not complete definitive surgical therapy by December 31, 2009, and those patients with cancers that did not fall within the American Joint Committee on Cancer (AJCC) staging guidelines.[17] Demographic, clinical, and treatment variables of patients were recorded, including age at diagnosis, race, sex, marital status, date of treatment, clinical and pathologic staging, type of surgery, and location of surgery. The clinicopathologic variables recorded included tumor malignancy type, tumor size, histologic subtype, location of tumor, nodal status, and metastatic status.

The study population included women diagnosed with AJCC stage 0, stage I, or stage II breast cancer, who had undergone either BCT or mastectomy. Clinical staging was used in decision making for classification of patients unless full pathologic staging was available. Breast conservation procedures included lumpectomy, quadrantectomy, partial mastectomy, and segmental mastectomy. Mastectomy procedures included simple (total) mastectomy, modified radical mastectomy, radical mastectomy, and bilateral mastectomy. Surgical treatment was categorized by the intent to treat. Patients who underwent BCT initially but later went on to have mastectomy as their definitive procedure were placed in the BCT category.

Descriptive statistics including either mean and standard deviations or counts and percentages were calculated. For data measured on the interval scale, the Student *t* test was used. If the data were ordinal or not normally distributed, the Wilcoxon rank sum test was used. For nominal data, the chi-square test or the Fisher exact test was used. SAS, version 9.2, was used for all analyses. A 2-tailed P value of less than .05 was considered statistically significant. A multivariate logistic regression, with whether a mastectomy or BCT was performed as the independent variable, was conducted to determine the selection criteria for mastectomy.

RESULTS

The tumor registry identified a total of 4799 patients diagnosed with breast carcinoma between 1999 and 2009, from which the authors took a sample of 1199 patients for their analysis (**Table 1**). However, 228 patients were excluded from the analysis (exclusion criteria included male patients; patients with stage III or stage IV breast cancer; patients who did not complete definitive surgery by December 31, 2009; and those who underwent surgical procedures other than BCT or mastectomy). Some of the patients met the criteria for more than 1 exclusion category. The remaining 971 patients were women with AJCC stage 0, stage I, or stage II breast carcinoma, who underwent BCT or mastectomy, and they were the study population for the analysis.

Patient and tumor characteristics of the study population are detailed in **Table 2**. BCT was performed in 75% of the patients. Mean age at diagnosis for the BCT group was 57.3 years compared with 54.1 years for the mastectomy group (range, 26–95 years; $P = .0008$). Postmenopausal women (older than 55 years) made up 55.2% of the BCT group. More than 78% of the total number of women older than 55 years underwent BCT as opposed to 71% of women younger than 55 years. The racial makeup in the BCT group was 81.7% white, 14.6% black, and 3.7% other ethnic categories. The mastectomy group had 82.5% white, 16.3% black, and 1.3% other ethnic categories. Most of the tumors in the BCT group were small (71.9% of cases vs 47.1% in the mastectomy group). Conversely, the mastectomy group had tumors that were predominantly in the larger size ranges; 47.6% in the 2 to 5 cm range and 5.2% in the larger than 5 cm group. Ductal tumors were the most represented histologic subtype in both the groups (78.8% in the BCT group and 76.7% in the mastectomy group). A histologic grade was assigned to 89.1% of cases, and 25.2% were well differentiated in the BCT group compared with 14.3% in the mastectomy group. Poorly differentiated tumors accounted for 39.2% of the mastectomy group. Stages 0 and I carcinomas were more common in the BCT group (combined total of 70% of cases) and represented only half of the cases in the mastectomy group.

A univariate analysis of patient and tumor characteristics in the study population was performed to determine the factors that may be predictive of BCT. Patients with favorable prognostic characteristics such as stage 0 or stage 1, less than 2 cm, and well-differentiated tumors were found to be positively associated with the likelihood of undergoing BCT. Postmenopausal women were found to be more likely to undergo BCT than mastectomy. Race and marital status were not found to be

Table 1
Characteristics of the 1199 patients comprising the study population

Characteristic	No. of Cases (%)
Sex	
Female	1186 (98.9)
Male	13 (1.1)
Menopausal status (age, y)	
<55	572 (47.7)
≥55	627 (52.3)
Race[a]	
White	950 (79.2)
Black	194 (16.1)
Other	16 (1.3)
Marital status[b]	
Single	156 (13.0)
Married	742 (62.0)
Separated/divorced	123 (10.3)
Widowed	136 (11.4)
Tumor size (cm)[c]	
<2	606 (61.3)
2–5	315 (31.9)
>5	67 (6.8)
Histologic subtype[d]	
Ductal	934 (78.0)
Lobular	83 (6.9)
Ductal and lobular	49 (4.1)
Mixed	30 (2.5)
Other	102 (8.5)
Location	
Upper outer quadrant	427 (35.6)
Upper inner quadrant	126 (10.5)
Lower outer quadrant	127 (10.6)
Lower inner quadrant	70 (5.8)
Central/nipple	47 (3.8)
Overlapping lesion	286 (23.9)
Other (NOS, axillary tail)	116 (9.7)
Grade[e]	
Well differentiated	207 (20.0)
Moderately differentiated	506 (48.9)
Poorly differentiated	321 (31.0)
AJCC stage[f]	
Stage 0	244 (21.2)
Stage I	463 (40.3)
Stage II	325 (28.2)
Stage III	88 (7.7)
Stage IV	29 (2.5)

Abbreviation: NOS, not otherwise specified.

[a] Not specified in 39 cases.
[b] Not specified in 3 cases.
[c] Not specified in 211 cases.
[d] Not specified in 1 case.
[e] Not specified in 163 cases.
[f] Not specified in 50 cases.

Table 2
Patient and tumor characteristics in the study population

Characteristic	No. of Cases		P Value
	BCT (%) (n = 721)	Mastectomy (%) (n = 240)	
Menopausal status (age, y)			
<55	323 (44.8)	132 (55.0)	.0061
≥55	398 (55.2)	108 (45.0)	
Mean age at diagnosis (y)	57.3	54.1	.0008
Race			
White	589 (81.7)	198 (82.5)	.1390
Black	105 (14.6)	39 (16.3)	
Other	27 (3.7)	3 (1.3)	
Marital status[a]			
Single	83 (11.5)	32 (13.4)	.0576
Married	461 (64.1)	150 (62.8)	
Separated/divorced	69 (9.6)	29 (12.1)	
Widowed	88 (12.2)	25 (10.5)	
Tumor size (cm)[b]			
≤2	455 (71.9)	99 (47.1)	<.0001
2–5	161 (25.4)	100 (47.6)	
>5	17 (2.7)	11 (5.2)	
Histologic subtype[c]			
Ductal	567 (78.8)	184 (76.7)	.04876
Lobular	45 (6.3)	19 (7.9)	
Ductal and lobular	28 (3.9)	13 (5.4)	
Mixed	17 (2.4)	8 (3.3)	
Other	63 (8.8)	16 (6.7)	
Location			
Upper outer quadrant	264 (36.6)	79 (32.9)	.6612
Upper inner quadrant	93 (12.9)	22 (9.2)	
Lower outer quadrant	78 (10.8)	32 (13.3)	
Lower inner quadrant	47 (6.5)	15 (6.3)	
Central/nipple	25 (3.5)	12 (5.0)	
Overlapping lesion	158 (21.9)	58 (24.2)	
Other (NOS, axillary tail)	56 (7.8)	22 (9.2)	
Grade[d]			
Well differentiated	161 (25.2)	31 (14.3)	<.0001
Moderately differentiated	317 (49.5)	101 (46.5)	
Poorly differentiated	162 (25.3)	85 (39.2)	
AJCC stage			
Stage 0	176 (24.4)	43 (17.9)	<.0001
Stage I	358 (49.6)	82 (34.2)	
Stage II	187 (25.9)	115 (47.9)	
Lymph node status			
Mean number of nodes examined	7.5	10.6	<.0001
Mean number of nodes positive	0.4	0.70	.0002

Abbreviation: NOS, not otherwise specified.
[a] Unknown or not specified in 24 cases.
[b] Not specified in 118 cases.
[c] Not specified in 1 case.
[d] Not specified in 104 cases.

significantly associated with either procedure. Location of tumor and histologic subtype did not show any significance. Positive lymph node status, regardless of the number of positive nodes, was found to be a predictor of mastectomy.

In the 11 years evaluated, there was a steady increase in the number of operations performed at CMC (**Fig. 1**, **Table 3**). The BCT rate increased from 65% in 1999 to 73.9% in 2009, with a peak rate of 87.7% in 2006. The mastectomy rate was cut by almost one-third, dropping from 35% in 1999 to 26% in 2009 (**Fig. 2**). The BCT rates at CMC in the years 2000 and 2008 were compared with those of both North Carolina and the United States. The BCT rate of 61% at CMC in 2000 was right at the national average of 62%, with North Carolina lagging behind at 54%. By 2008, the rates of BCT had increased to 78%, 64%, and 59%, respectively, with North Carolina BCT rate still less than the national average.[18]

A logistic regression model was used to determine if any of the factors found to be statistically significant were independently predictive of BCT (**Table 4**). Among the tumor characteristics, only tumor size remained statistically significant after inclusion into the regression model. Women with tumor size less than 2 cm had a 50% less chance of undergoing mastectomy than women with larger tumors. Those patients with positive lymph nodes were 1.7 times as likely to undergo mastectomy compared with patients with a negative nodal status (95% confidence interval, 1.101–2.906). Stage, menopausal status, and grade did not remain significant after inclusion into the regression model.

DISCUSSION

BCT was proved to have equivalent survival rates compared with mastectomy in several large prospectively randomized studies with 20-year follow-up data.[1,2] Based on these findings, guidelines for the treatment of early-stage breast cancer were published in 1990 that promoted BCT as an appropriate treatment modality for these patients.[19] Although variations in the rate of adoption of a new procedure are not uncommon, the treatment of early-stage breast cancer with BCT has been surprisingly slow to increase despite strong evidence from randomized trials.

Initial rates of BCT were found to be quite low in some studies, but varied depending on the data source and geographic location evaluated. In a 1986 study using the Medicare data of 36,982 women, Nattinger and colleagues[5] found a BCT rate of 12%. Substantial regional variation was also seen with a rate as low as 3.5% in Kentucky

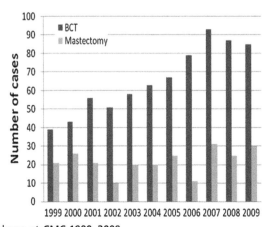

Fig. 1. Surgical volume at CMC 1999–2009.

Table 3 Number of surgeries by year			
	No. of Surgeries (%)		
Year	BCT	Mastectomy	Total
1999	39 (65.0)	21 (35.0)	60
2000	43 (62.3)	26 (37.7)	69
2001	56 (72.7)	21 (27.3)	77
2002	51 (83.6)	10 (16.4)	61
2003	58 (74.4)	20 (25.6)	78
2004	63 (75.9)	20 (24.1)	83
2005	67 (72.8)	25 (27.2)	92
2006	79 (87.8)	11 (12.2)	90
2007	93 (75.0)	31 (25.0)	124
2008	87 (77.7)	25 (22.3)	112
2009	85 (73.9)	30 (26.1)	115
Total	721	240	961

to as high as 21.2% in Massachusetts. North Carolina was at the lower end of the spectrum with a rate of 4.8%. A follow-up study comparing rates from 1986 to 1990 found only a minimal increase in the BCT rate, up to 15%, whereas regional variation in BCT rates remained persistent.[20] These studies may underestimate the actual BCT rates because they sampled an older patient population, a factor consistently found to be associated with higher rates of mastectomies. A more recent study using a Medicare database surveyed 56,725 women treated for breast cancer in 2001 and found a BCT rate of 59% versus a 41% mastectomy rate.[21] A Department of Defense (DoD) study of the treatment of early-stage breast cancer between 1986 and 1996 observed an increase in BCT from 16% to 47%.[13] Interestingly, regional variation in BCT rates was also observed within the DoD health care system, despite the routine availability of radiation therapy and the regularity with which military surgeons on active duty move between regions and hospital types. The investigators postulated

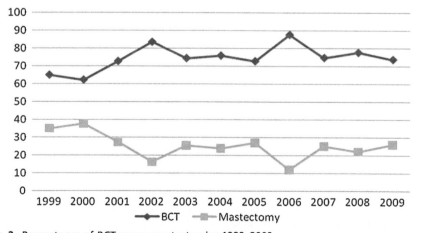

Fig. 2. Percentages of BCT versus mastectomies 1999–2009.

Table 4
Multivariate analysis of clinicopathologic predictors of BCT

Selected Characteristic	Adjusted Odds Ratio	95% Confidence Interval	P Value
Age >55 y	0.761	0.561–1.032	.0790
Tumor size <2 cm	0.500	0.340–0.736	.0004[a]
Grade (well differentiated)	0.659	0.429–1.012	.0566
AJCC stage	1.183	0.715–1.956	.5127
Any positive node	1.789	1.101–2.906	.0249[a]

[a] P value demonstrates statistical significance.

that perhaps an adoption of regional attitudes by patients in the treatment groups may have accounted for the observed regional variation. Large national databases are conducive for determining BCT rates across the country, but they are limited by both the type of information included in the data and the patient population itself, and may not be reflective of the true BCT rate.

Wide variation in BCT rates has also been demonstrated in several studies that have looked at BCT rates within a single state or hospital system. Guadagnoli and colleagues[20] identified patients at almost 50 randomly selected hospitals in 2 states between 1983 and 1985 and reported different rates of breast conservation. The investigators found that in Massachusetts, 74% of women eligible for breast conservation underwent BCT, whereas 48% did so in Minnesota. A Connecticut study found an overall BCT rate of 57.7% during the period 1991 to 1995, along with geographic variation of treatment within the state.[21] These studies have certain limitations because of the smaller population sizes examined but remain useful in comparisons with other similar communities.

In the authors' sample of women treated for breast carcinoma at CMC, we found an overall BCT rate of 75%, with 78% in 2008. Compared with the 2008 data from the National Cancer Data Base, the CMC rate was higher than the national average of 64% and substantially more than the rate of 59% for North Carolina (**Fig. 3**). There may be some overestimation of the true BCT rate at CMC because of unintentional over-sampling of patients who underwent BCT. A review of the entire data set may answer this question. The BCT rate at CMC may also be higher than that in North Carolina because it is an academic community hospital located in an urban setting and may

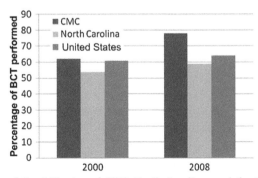

Fig. 3. Comparison of the BCT rates of CMC, North Carolina, and the United States. (*Data from* The National Cancer Data Base. Available at: http://cromwell.facs.org/BMarks/BMPub/Ver10/bm_reports.cfm. Accessed October 1, 2010.)

be more similar to other urban medical centers than to many of the hospitals in the rest of the state. A study conducted by Answini and colleagues[22] compared BCT rates from 1995 to 1997 between the Charlotte-Mecklenburg county and 6 surrounding rural counties in North Carolina. They found statistically significant higher rates of BCT in the former than the latter for both stage I (59% vs 42%) and stage II (37% and 19%, respectively) cancers. In our study evaluating the same urban setting 10 years later, BCT rates were found to be higher but remained consistent with the findings in the earlier study by Answini and colleagues. The higher rate seen in our study may also be reflective of surgeons in Charlotte using BCT more frequently than in the past, coupled with more frequent use of neoadjuvant chemotherapy. The increasing use of Internet may have a contributing role in the increase in breast conservation because many patients are now highly educated about their disease and the possible treatment options. Contrary to this theory, one study found that greater patient involvement in treatment decisions was associated with a greater likelihood of mastectomy.[23] A more comprehensive look at the CMC database may be able to explain why the authors' sample demonstrated a greater percentage of BCT in postmenopausal women, a finding dissimilar to that seen in numerous other studies.[4,6,7,14]

With current nationwide efforts moving toward pay-for-performance and the resulting creation of centers of excellence, the question then becomes, "Can BCT be a suitable benchmark to measure quality of care?" Initial quality measures for breast cancer were put forth in 2007 by a collaborative group of cancer networks (the Commission on Cancer, the American Society of Clinical Oncology, and the National Comprehensive Cancer Network) and then endorsed by the National Quality Forum. These measures addressed the following: ideal timing of radiation therapy, consideration or administration of chemotherapy, and consideration or administration of tamoxifen or other third-generation aromatase inhibitors within 1 year of diagnosis in those patients who met the criteria for receiving these therapies.[24] Although breast conservation is not indicated for every patient with early-stage breast cancer, it may be able to serve as a quality indicator for nationally accepted standards of care in cancer treatment. Further research on the role that breast conservation may provide in reflecting standards of care would be useful in providing the answer to the aforementioned question.

SUMMARY

Despite strong evidence supporting the use of BCT, actual rates of BCT use remain lower than expected. Geographic variation persists, with lower rates particularly in the south. This article is a retrospective review of a sample of patients from the hospital cancer registry comparing BCT and mastectomy rates during an 11-year period. BCT rates have increased in CMC over this time frame and have reached national levels. Further research is needed to determine whether these rates can be used as a benchmark for care of the patients with cancer.

ACKNOWLEDGMENTS

The authors would like to thank Sharon Gilkerson from the Carolinas Medical Center Cancer Registry for her help in this study.

REFERENCES

1. Veronesi U, Cascinelli N, Mariani L, et al. Twenty year follow-up of a randomized study comparing breast-conserving surgery with radical mastectomy for early breast cancer. N Engl J Med 2002;347(16):1227–32.

2. Fisher B, Anderson S, Bryant J, et al. Twenty year follow-up of a randomized trial comparing total mastectomy, lumpectomy, and lumpectomy plus irradiation for the treatment of invasive breast cancer. N Engl J Med 2002;347(16):1233–41.

3. Morrow M, Khan S. Breast disease. In: Mulholland MW, Lillemoe KD, Doherty GM, et al, editors. Greenfield's surgery: scientific principles and practice. 4th edition. Philadelphia: Lippincott Williams & Wilkins; 2006. p. 1251–89.

4. Farrow DC, Hunt WC, Samet JM. Geographic variation in the treatment of localized breast cancer. N Engl J Med 1992;326:1097–101.

5. Nattinger AB, Gottlier MS, Veum J, et al. Geographic variation in the use of breast-conserving treatment for breast cancer. N Engl J Med 1992;326(17): 1102–7.

6. Lazovich D, White E, Thomas D, et al. Underutilization of breast-conserving surgery and radiation therapy among women with stage I or II breast cancer. JAMA 1991;266(24):3433–8.

7. Johantgen ME, Coffey RM, Harris DR, et al. Treating early-stage breast cancer: hospital characteristics associated with breast-conserving surgery. Am J Public Health 1995;85(10):1432–4.

8. Gilligan MA, Neuner J, Sparapani R, et al. Surgeon characteristics and variations in treatment for early-stage breast cancer. Arch Surg 2007;142:17–22.

9. Voti L, Richardson LC, Reis IM, et al. Treatment of local breast carcinoma in Florida. Cancer 2005;106(1):201–7.

10. Morrow M, Jagsi R, Alderman AK, et al. Surgeon recommendations and receipt of mastectomy for treatment of breast cancer. JAMA 2009;302(14):1551–6.

11. Smith GL, Xu Y, Shih YT, et al. Breast-conserving surgery in older patients with invasive breast cancer: current patterns of treatment across the United States. J Am Coll Surg 2009;209(4):425–33.

12. McGuire KP, Santillan AA, Kaur P, et al. Are mastectomies on the rise? A 13-year trend analysis of the selection of mastectomy versus breast conservation therapy in 5865 patients. Ann Surg Oncol 2009;16:2682–90.

13. Kelemen JJ, Poulton T, Swartz M, et al. Surgical treatment of early-stage breast cancer in the Department of Defense healthcare system. J Am Coll Surg 2001; 192:293–7.

14. Morrow M, White J, Moughan J, et al. Factors predicting the use of breast-conserving therapy in stage I and II breast carcinoma. J Clin Oncol 2001;19(8): 2254–62.

15. Osteen RT, Steele GD Jr, Menck HR, et al. Regional differences in surgical management of breast cancer. CA Cancer J Clin 1992;42(1):39–43.

16. American Joint Committee on Cancer. AJCC cancer staging manual. 6th edition. New York: Springer-Verlag; 2002.

17. Data from National Cancer Database. Commission on Cancer Website. Available at: http://cromwell.facs.org/BMarks/BMPub/Ver10/bm_reports.cfm. Accessed October 7, 2010.

18. NIH Consensus Conference. Treatment of early-stage breast cancer. JAMA 1991; 265(3):391–5.

19. Nattinger AB, Gottlieb MS, Hoffman RG, et al. Minimal increase in use of breast-conserving surgery from 1986–1990. Med Care 1996;34(5):479–89.

20. Guadagnoli E, Weeks JC, Shapiro JH, et al. Use of breast-conserving surgery for treatment of stage I and stage II breast cancer. J Clin Oncol 1998;16(1): 101–6.

21. Gregorio DI, Kulldorff M, Barry L, et al. Geographical differences in primary therapy for early-stage breast cancer. Ann Surg Oncol 2001;8(10):844–9.

22. Answini GA, Woodard WL, Norton HJ, et al. Breast conservation: trends in a major southern metropolitan area compared with surrounding rural counties. Am Surg 2001;67:994–8.
23. Katz SJ, Lantz PM, Janz NK, et al. Patient involvement in surgery treatment decisions for breast cancer. J Clin Oncol 2005;23(24):5526–33.
24. News from the American College of Surgeons. ACS web site. Available at: http://www.facs.org/news/qc-cancer.html. Accessed October 9, 2010.

American College of Surgeons Oncology Group and the Community Surgeon

David M. Ota, MD[a],*, A. Marilyn Leitch, MD[b], Gary Unzeitig, MD[c]

KEYWORDS

- American College of Surgeons Oncology Group
- Community surgeon • Oncology • Cancer trials

The American College of Surgeons Oncology Group (ACOSOG) conducts cancer trials that are relevant to surgeons who treat patients with breast, thoracic, and gastrointestinal cancers. ACOSOG is funded by the National Cancer Institute and is charged with conducting prospective clinical trials that address important questions in both academic and community practice settings. Examples include role of axillary dissection for microscopic nodal disease, neoadjuvant therapy for organ-conserving surgery, laparoscopic rectal cancer resection, mediastinal nodal staging, and sublobar resection for early-stage non–small cell lung cancer (NSCLC). Such trials are relevant to most practicing surgeons.

ACOSOG was established in 1999 as a national surgeon-based clinical trial cooperative group. Early on, the scientific leadership that developed the trials consisted of surgeons but has evolved to include medical oncologists, radiation oncologists, radiologists, and pathologists. Because cancer treatment is multidisciplinary, current ACOSOG trials have multiple treatment combinations while retaining a surgical focus.

There are several reasons for academic and community surgeons to participate in national clinical trials. First, resectable cancers are commonly seen in community practices and completion of a trial is best accomplished with both academic and community surgeon involvement. There are other reasons for community surgeons to participate in clinical trials. Surgeons are tasked with improving the outcomes of surgical patients. New instruments, procedures, and therapeutic agents are a constant feature of our innovative medical culture, and community surgeons involved in trials

[a] Department of Surgery, Duke University, 2400 Pratt Street, Terrace Level, Room 0311, Durham, NC 27705, USA
[b] University of Texas Medical Center, 5323 Harry Hines Boulevard, Dallas, TX 75390, USA
[c] Doctors Hospital of Laredo, 10700 McPherson Road, Laredo, TX 78045, USA
* Corresponding author.
E-mail address: david.ota@duke.edu

Surg Oncol Clin N Am 20 (2011) 439–445
doi:10.1016/j.soc.2011.01.006
1055-3207/11/$ – see front matter © 2011 Elsevier Inc. All rights reserved.

surgonc.theclinics.com

are most likely to keep current with new technology. Furthermore, prospective trials are essential to determine safety and outcome of a new procedure or treatment. Lastly, participation in a clinical trial not only improves medical knowledge but also can enhance a surgeon's leadership in the community.[1] This can result in recognition as a leader in the medical community and as an advocate for science. ACOSOG recognizes the importance of community surgeons and has started to fill its scientific leadership positions with these surgeons.

A review of ACOSOG trials reveals that these studies have had an impact on surgical practice patterns and patient outcomes. The portfolio of trials is organized according to organ site and assigned to committees, including breast, gastrointestinal, and thoracic committees. Committee members include practicing surgeons, medical oncologists, radiation oncologists, statisticians, nurses/clinical research associates, and patient advocates. The committees are tasked with developing, assessing feasibility of, prioritizing, overseeing the conduct of, and promoting accrual to ACOSOG trials.

The ACOSOG breast committee has focused on important procedural and multidisciplinary cancer trials. The introduction of lymphatic mapping and sentinel lymph node (SLN) biopsy by Giuliano and associates[2,3] was a major advance in breast cancer surgery and has led to other important practice-changing trials. The most notable example is ACOSOG Z0011, the phase III randomized trial of axillary lymph node dissection versus SLN dissection alone for microscopic detected lymph node metastases. For more than a century, Halsted axillary dissection has been a standard surgical procedure for breast cancer.[4] The advent of lymphatic mapping and sentinel node biopsy changed surgical management of the axilla for breast cancer and melanoma. ACOSOG Z0011 showed no difference in local-regional control and overall survival between the two axillary procedures at 5-year follow-up.[5] This practice-changing trial provided data disputing the need for axillary dissection in patients who have less than or equal to 2 SLNs containing microscopic metastatic disease undergoing breast-conserving surgery (BCS) with radiation.

The breast committee conducted the Z0010 trial to assess the prognostic significance of micrometastases in the SLNs and bone marrow identified by immunohistochemistry (IHC) among patients presenting with clinical stage I and II disease. The focused examination of SLNs encouraged the application of IHC technology for detection of micrometastases when routine hematoxylin-eosin staining was negative for metastatic disease. The clinical significance of IHC-detected micrometastases and the implications for postoperative adjuvant therapy have not been clear. The Z0010 trial showed no difference in local and systemic recurrence rates in patients with SLN micrometastases compared with IHC-negative SLN subjects.[6] Trial data negate the value of routine IHC examination of SLNs in early-stage breast cancer. These two large trials required broad participation for their success.[7] Cancer surgery is primarily done in the private-practice setting, and enrollment to trials, such as these, require the involvement of all surgeons.

SLN trials are continuing. The legacy SLN trials (Z0010 and Z0011) involved early-stage disease. There has been substantial controversy, however, about the role of SLN biopsy in locally advanced breast cancer (LABC). Patients with LABC are often treated with neoadjuvant therapy with downstaging of the primary tumor and involved axillary lymph nodes. ACOSOG Z1071 (Study Chair Dr Judy Boughey) is a 660-patient phase II study of lymphatic mapping for patients who receive neoadjuvant chemotherapy for LABC with positive axillary lymph nodes confirmed by needle biopsy.[8] The primary objective is to determine the accuracy of lymphatic mapping and SLN biopsy after neoadjuvant chemotherapy in predicting residual nodal disease. Patients receive neoadjuvant chemotherapy and then undergo SLN biopsy and axillary lymph node dissection. This trial is rapidly accruing 40 patients a month and enrollment will be complete by November 2011. In keeping with the theme of minimizing surgical therapy, ACOSOG has undertaken a trial to look at another alternative primary tumor therapy. The Z1072 trial (Study Chair Dr Rache Simmons) involves cryoablation of less than 2-cm primary breast cancers, followed by MRI to assess for residual disease. Lumpectomy is then performed to histologically assess for residual viable tumor. If the postablation MRI proves to successfully document complete tumor ablation in this highly selected patient population, then larger randomized trials will be undertaken to validate ablation without surgical resection.

The breast committee is also conducting neoadjuvant systemic therapeutic trials for LABC to improve BCS rates. Z1031 (Study Chair Dr Matthew Ellis) is actively enrolling postmenopausal patients with clinical stage II or III palpable estrogen receptor (ER)-positive breast cancers. Instead of chemotherapy, patients receive neoadjuvant aromatase inhibitor (AI) for 16 weeks. The results of cohort A, 377 patients, were first reported at the American Society of Clinical Oncology 2010 annual meeting (ASCO 2010).[9] The clinical response to AI therapy was 60%. Those patients judged by their surgeons to be candidates for BCS before neoadjuvant AI therapy had an 85% BCS rate. There were 150 patients judged to require mastectomy and, after neoadjuvant AI therapy, 51% were converted to BCS. These are promising results, but the investigators are not satisfied with a 51% BCS rate. The study revealed that there is a subset of patients with highly ER-positive tumors who did not respond to AI therapy. This indicates that there is another mechanism or proliferative growth pathway overcoming the antiendocrine therapy. In cohort B of Z1031, a marker of proliferation, Ki67, is being analyzed in specimens from pretreatment biopsy and from a second biopsy at 2 weeks to select patents most likely to respond to AI for continuation of therapy. Those with an elevated Ki67 (>20%) after 2 weeks of AI therapy are switched to chemotherapy with the goal of assessing pathologic response in this selected patient population. Correlative science studies are ongoing to identify other predicators of AI resistance to improve the BCS rate.

Critical to the success of Z1031 is the ability of surgeons to acquire a research core needle biopsy of the palpable primary tumor before AI therapy is started and during the course of therapy. The specimen is frozen and sent to the ACOSOG tumor bank for RNA and DNA analysis. There is an emerging technology of whole genome sequencing of the tumor DNA looking for mutations of proliferative pathway genes.[10] Specific mutations in KIT, BRAF, and EGFR genes result in susceptibility to specific oral kinase inhibitors and are good examples of how DNA sequencing can detect gene mutations and direct targeted therapy. Remarkable laboratory investigation is only possible with the acquisition of well-preserved specimens of primary tumor. Every day, surgeons are resecting primary tumors and have the ability to acquire fresh tumor tissue for DNA analysis.

Z1041 (Study Chair Dr Aman Buzdar) addresses the use of targeted trastuzumab-anthracycline therapy for LABC that is HER2neu positive.[11] In a pilot study of this regimen, pathologic complete response (pCR) rates were as high as 65%.[12] In this randomized trial, the initial regimen is compared with a similar regimen in which trastuzumab is not given concurrently with 5-fluorouracil, epirubicin, and cyclophosphamide (FEC) to compare efficacy for pCR and variance in toxicity. The rate of BCS will be assessed and correlative studies will assess for markers to chemosensitivity.

The gastrointestinal committee trial portfolio includes studies addressing surgical issues, adjuvant therapy, and neoadjuvant approaches for minimizing surgical intervention. Z9001 (Study Chair Dr Ron DeMatteo) is a phase III, double-blind, randomized adjuvant trial of placebo versus imatinib for resected gastrointestinal stromal tumors (GISTs). This trial opened in 2001 and completed accrual of 713 evaluable patients in 2007. There were considerable concerns about the feasibility of completing this trial when only 5000 new GIST cases per year are diagnosed in the United States. In 2001, the National Cancer Data Base was queried to identify hospitals with a high volume of GIST patients; it was discovered that there were no high-volume sites. GIST is treated by community surgeons. The trial enrolled 717 GIST subjects from 234 sites. Although GIST is an uncommon cancer, surgical resection and investigational targeted therapy can be done in a community setting. Without a large number of participating sites, this first adjuvant trial of a novel targeted agent would not have been possible. The Z9001 GIST adjuvant trial shows that when a trial asks a scientifically important question, there is broad participation. This trial also emphasized that a clinical trial must have impact on clinical practices and therein lays the importance of the science to practicing surgeons.[13]

The gastrointestinal committee has conducted neoadjuvant trials that facilitate minimally invasive surgical procedures. Z6041 (Study Chair Dr Julio Garcia-Aguilar) is a completed phase II trial of neoadjuvant chemoradiation therapy followed by local excision of T1N0M0 rectal carcinomas less than 4 cm. The early results of the trials were reported at ASCO 2010.[14] One objective of this study is to assess the pCR rate in resected specimens. There were 79 evaluable patients with a 43% pCR. An R0 resection with local excision was achieved in 98% of patients. A significant limitation of the oxaliplatin-capecitabine radiation therapy, however, was its toxicity. Thus, a successor trial is in development with the objective of reducing the toxicity of the neoadjuvant regimen while maintaining a high pCR rate.

Mutational analysis of the primary tumor biopsy specimens from Z6041 is currently being done. There is considerable interest in KRAS mutation and radiotherapy resistance. The objective of these analyses is to develop a predictive model for pCR using mutation analysis of KRAS, other proliferative pathway genes, or DNA repair genes. Such investigations may give clues to select targeted agents that maximize tumor downstaging to achieve an R0 local excision for early rectal cancer.

The gastrointestinal committee is committed to prospectively assessing novel surgical procedures. Z6051 (Study Chair Dr James Fleshman) is a phase III trial comparing laparoscopic-assisted resection with open resection for rectal cancer. A major quality indicator for rectal cancer resection is total mesorectal excision (TME). TME requires an intact mesorectum and covering peritoneal envelope to the level of rectal transection with no coning in of the mesorectum above the point of transection. This trial will determine if laparoscopic-assisted resection is not inferior to open rectal resection based on (1) circumferential margin, (2) distal margin, and (3) completeness of TME. This trial is open and has enrolled 206 patients with a monthly accrual rate of 9 patients a month. The accrual goal is 480 patients with an estimated completion date of May 2013.

The thoracic committee has been actively involved with trials that focus on accurate early lung cancer staging, resection techniques for stage 1 disease, and locally advanced esophageal adenocarcinoma. Z30 (Study Chair Dr Mark Allen) is a phase III trial comparing mediastinal lymph node dissection with mediastinal lymph node sampling for T1N0N1 NSCLC. This trial enrolled 1111 patients in fewer than 5 years. In 2006, Allen and colleagues[15] published the perioperative outcomes for the two mediastinal nodal staging procedures. There were no differences in hospital length of stay, chest tube days, and complications. Darling and colleagues[16] recently reported that at 6.3-year follow-up there was no difference in survival between the two mediastinal nodal staging procedures.

An important clinical question in thoracic surgical oncology is risk of local recurrence after a sublobar resection for T1 NSCLC in those patients who are not candidates for lobectomy because of the higher risk of complications. Local recurrence could be as high as 20%. Z4032 (Study Chair Dr Hiran Fernando) is a phase III trial comparing sublobar resection with sublobar resection plus brachytherapy. The hypothesis states that radiation seeds placed over the staple line of the sublobar resection reduce local recurrence.[17] The primary objective is to determine local recurrence rates between the two treatment arms. The trial completed accrual of 227 patients in early 2010 and follow-up continues for recurrence. Fernando and colleagues[18,19] recently reported that brachytherapy did not adversely affect postoperative pulmonary function or dyspnea scores.[20]

The scientific questions of ACOSOG trials are encountered in everyday practice. These questions are relevant to practicing surgeons. Community surgeons contribute to 40% of ACOSOG enrollment. Although the legacy trials focused on surgical procedures, the current trials are more multidisciplinary, demonstrating the maturity of ACOSOG and its network of oncologists in all specialties. Because ACOSOG trials focus on early disease and surgical management questions, these trials should appeal to all surgeons. These trials have demonstrated surgeons' ability to acquire fresh tissue at the time of surgery for central specimen bank storage. Surgeons in both community and academic settings have been highly successful in fresh tissue acquisition, which is critical to ACOSOG research aims. Surgeons have taken on the complex task of obtaining informed consent for tissue acquisition for laboratory investigations, such as DNA sequencing, and, because they evaluate patients with resectable disease, they are able to answer questions and reassure patients that their privacy will be protected in these investigations.

ACOSOG has worked diligently to provide a broad portfolio of trials that is relevant to practicing surgeons who treat breast, gastrointestinal, and thoracic malignancies. The ACOSOG Web site provides information about membership, meetings, and protocols. This is research for practicing surgeons who are committed to improving the treatment of their cancer patients. These trials require surgeon leadership to successfully accrue patients who have early-stage disease. Surgeons must decide to offer their patients participation in prospective clinical trials to advance surgical knowledge.

REFERENCES

1. Unzeitig G. How a surgeon in the boonies becomes a researcher and regional expert. Bull Am Coll Surg 2007;92(12):33–4.
2. Giuliano AE, Kirgan DM, Guenther JM, et al. Lymphatic mapping and sentinel lymphadenectomy for breast cancer. Ann Surg 1994;220(3):391–401 [discussion: 8–401].
3. Giuliano AE, Jones RC, Brennan M, et al. Sentinel lymphadenectomy in breast cancer. J Clin Oncol 1997;26(6):2345–50.
4. Halsted WS. I. The results of radical operations for the cure of carcinoma of the breast. Ann Surg 1907;46(1):1–19.
5. Giuliano A, McCall L, Beitsch P, et al. Locoregional recurrence after sentinel lymph node dissection with or without axillary dissection in patients with sentinel lymph node metastases: the American college of surgeons oncology group Z0011 randomized trial. Ann Surg 2010;252:426–32 [discussion: 32–3].
6. Cote RJ, Giuliano AE, Hawes D, et al. ACOSOG Z0010. A multicenter prognostic study of sentinel node (SN) and bone marrow (BM) micrometastases in women with clinical T1/T2 N0 M0 breast cancer. ASCO; 2010. Best of ASCO 2010;28:18s.

7. Leitch AM, Beitsch PD, McCall LM, et al. Patterns of participation and successful patient recruitment to American College of Surgeons Oncology Group Z0010, a phase II trial for patients with early-stage breast cancer. Am J Surg 2005; 190(4):539–42.

8. Boughey JC, Hunt K, Le-Petross HT, et al. A phase II study evaluating the role of sentinel lymph node surgery and axillary lymph node dissection following preoperative chemotherapy in women with node-positive breast cancer (T1–4, N1-2, M0) at initial diagnosis: ACOSOG Z1071. ASCO; 2010. Available at: http://www. asco.org/ASCOv2/Meetings/Abstracts?&vmview=abst_detail_view&confID=74& abstractID=41100; http://meeting.ascopubs.org/cgi/content/abstract/28/15_suppl/ TPS118. Accessed June, 2010.

9. Ellis MJ, Buzdar AU, Unzeitig GW, et al. ACOSOG Z1031. A randomized phase III trial comparing exemestane, letrozole and anastrozole in postmenopausal women with clinical stage 2/3 estrogen receptor positive breast cancer. ASCO; 2010. Available at: http://abstract.asco.org/AbstView_74_47842.html. Accessed June, 2010.

10. Ding L, Ellis MJ, Li S, et al. Genome remodelling in a basal-like breast cancer metastasis and xenograft. Nature 2010;464(7291):999–1005.

11. Buzdar AU, Ballman KV, Meric-Bernstam F, et al. Preliminary safety data of a randomized phase III trial comparing a preoperative regimen of FEC-75 alone followed by paclitaxel plus trastuzumab with a regimen of paclitaxel plus trastuzumab followed by FEC-75 plus trastuzumab in patients with HER2 positive operable breast cancer (ACOSOG Z1041). ASCO Annual Meeting. Chicago (IL), June, 2010.

12. Buzdar AU, Ibrahim NK, Francis D, et al. Significantly higher pathologic complete remission rate after neoadjuvant therapy with trastuzumab, paclitaxel, and epirubicin chemotherapy: results of a randomized trial in human epidermal growth factor receptor 2-positive operable breast cancer. J Clin Oncol 2005;23(16): 3676–85.

13. DeMatteo RP, Ballman KV, Antonescu CR, et al. Adjuvant imatinib mesylate after resection of localised, primary gastrointestinal stromal tumour: a randomised, double-blind, placebo-controlled trial. Lancet 2009;373(9669):1097–104.

14. Garcia-Aguilar J, Shi Q, Thomas CR, et al. Pathologic complete response (pCR) to neoadjuvant chemoradiation (CRT) and local excision (LE) for uT2uN0 rectal cancer (RC): results of the ACOSOG Z6041 trial. ASCO; 2010. Available at: http://www.asco.org/ASCOv2/Meetings/Abstracts?&vmview=abst_detail_view& confID=74&abstractID=51920; http://meeting.ascopubs.org/cgi/content/abstract/ 28/15_suppl/3510. Accessed June, 2010.

15. Allen MS, Darling GE, Pechet TT, et al. Morbidity and mortality of major pulmonary resections in patients with early-stage lung cancer: initial results of the randomized, prospective ACOSOG Z0030 trial. Ann Thorac Surg 2006;81(3):1013–9 [discussion: 9–20].

16. Darling G, Allen MS, Decker PA, et al. Randomized trial of mediastinal lymph node sampling versus complete lymphadenectomy during pulmonary resection in the patient with N0 or N1 (Less Than Hilar) non-small cell carcinoma: results of the ACOSOG Z0030 trial. American Association of Thoracic Surgery; 2010. Available at: http://www.aats.org/annualmeeting/Abstracts/2010/1.html. Accessed May, 2010.

17. Smith RP, Schuchert M, Komanduri K, et al. Dosimetric evaluation of radiation exposure during I-125 vicryl mesh implants: implications for ACOSOG Z4032. Ann Surg Oncol 2007;14(12):3610–3.

18. Fernando HC, Landreneau R, Mandraker S, et al. The impact of adjuvant brachytherapy with sublobar resection on pulmonary function and dyspnea in high-risk operable patients: preliminary results form the ACOSOG Z4032 trial. J Thorac Cardiovasc Surg 2011. in press.

19. Fernando HC, Landreneau R, Mandraker S, et al. The impact of adjuvant brachytherapy with sublobar resection on pulmonary function and dyspnea: preliminary results from ACOSOG Z4032 trial. American Association Thoracic Surgery; 2010. Available at: http://www.aats.org/annualmeeting/Abstracts/2010/15.html. Accessed May, 2010.

20. Fernando HC, Landrenau RJ, Mandraker S, et al. Thirty and ninety day outcomes after sublobar resection of high-risk patients with non-small cell lung cancer [NSCLC]; results from a multicenter phase III study. J Thorac Cardiovasc Surg, in press.

A Community Hospital Clinical Trials Program: Infrastructure for Growth

Louis H. Barr, MD[a],*, Jane Crofton, RN, BSN, OCN, CCRP[b],
Yu-Hsin Annie Lin, MD[c]

KEYWORDS

- Clinical trials • Community hospital • Tumor boards
- Patient care navigators

This article (1) reviews the experience of a clinical trials program at a large community hospital; (2) presents the growth of our trials program along with the increasing number of site-specific tumor boards; and (3) also examines the role of clinical care coordinators, often referred to as patient care navigators. By coordinating and directing patients along a path of optimal multidisciplinary evaluation including presentation at appropriate tumor boards, the authors believe there has been increased participation in clinical trials. They also believe these 2 modalities go hand-in-hand in providing an infrastructure needed to maintain and grow an active community hospital clinical trials program.

DEVELOPMENT OF CLINICAL TRIALS PROGRAMS

Clinical trials hold the key to treatment decisions in medicine by bringing basic science research and clinical advances to the mainstream of clinical practice. They have provided a means of translating what we learn in the laboratory into the clinic and build an ever-expanding knowledge base and experience. The role of clinical trials is particularly unique in oncology clinical research. The authors often explain to the residents that to know and understand the early advances in breast cancer

The authors have nothing to disclose.
[a] Florida Hospital Cancer Institute, Florida Hospital, 2501 North Orange Avenue, Suite 289, Orlando, FL 32804, USA
[b] Florida Hospital Cancer Institute, Florida Hospital, 2501 North Orange Avenue, Suite 683, Orlando, FL 32804, USA
[c] General Surgery Residency, Florida Hospital, 2501 North Orange Avenue, Suite 301, Orlando, FL 32804, USA
* Corresponding author.
E-mail address: louis.barr.md@flhosp.org

Surg Oncol Clin N Am 20 (2011) 447–453
doi:10.1016/j.soc.2011.01.001
1055-3207/11/$ – see front matter © 2011 Elsevier Inc. All rights reserved.

treatment, one could study the progression and outcomes of the National Surgical Adjuvant Breast Project clinical trials starting from the 1970s. These trials were somewhat unique in that they included both drug protocols and surgical procedures. The application of these trials, along with others such as from the Milan National Cancer Institute (NCI) by Dr Veronesi has been critical in advancing cancer treatment.[1] In more recent years, the American College of Surgeons Oncology Group (ACOSOG) has also become active in bringing more surgery-related studies to the participating community surgeon as well.

Up to 30 years ago, 80% of clinical trials were done in the academic setting in spite of 80% to 85% of cancer patients being under the care of community oncologists.[2] In 1983, the NCI started the Community Clinical Oncology Program (CCOP) in which community and private physician participation was encouraged. By 1994, Fleming[3] reported that the number of clinical trials done in the community had increased to 60%, with 40% in academic or dedicated cancer centers. In that same year, Cobau[4] reported almost one-third of all patients on clinical trials were accrued via the CCOP program. Though there were initial quality concerns, there proved to be no difference in patient evaluability, eligibility, morbidity, or mortality These concerns were also examined more recently by Wilke and colleagues[5] when looking at National Quality Forum performance measures for breast cancer treatment in the ACOSOG Z0010 breast trial. Data were reviewed from teaching affiliated, academic, and community hospitals. This multiinstitutional trial found excellent compliance with the quality standards regardless of practice environment. This finding was also supported by Lamont and colleagues.[6] They reviewed outcomes from phase III Cancer and Leukemia Group B (CALGB) lung cancer trials at 272 different treatment sites, including academic centers, community hospitals, and Veteran Hospital Administration affiliates. There was no difference in patient survival that could be related to the enrollment setting. They also found that patients enrolled in the community setting provided an important heterogeneity, thus making such studies more relevant to general practice.

Clinical trial participation has been encouraged by many organizations including the American Society of Clinical Oncology (ASCO), the Society of Surgical Oncology, and the National Comprehensive Cancer Network. When following National Comprehensive Cancer Network (NCCN) guidelines, a statement is made for each tumor site: "the NCCN believes the best management of any cancer patient is in a clinical trial. Participation in clinical trials is especially encouraged." An editorial by Burstein[7] when discussing the comprehensive nature of the NCCN guidelines states that "this thoroughness creates somewhat of an illusion, however, that NCCN guidelines panel members always know the right thing to do next, that little uncertainty exists, or that things couldn't be done better. This is rarely the case in oncology, of course, which is why clinical trials are needed."

Participation in clinical trials is considered a measure of a cancer program's success. Clinical trial accrual is an important eligibility criterion for participation and accreditation with the American College of Surgeons Commission on Cancer.[8] A Comprehensive Community Hospital Cancer Program designation requires 2% of annual newly diagnosed cancer patients to be accrued. This percentage of cancer patients increases to 4% for a Teaching Hospital Program and 6% for Network Cancer Program designation.

In spite of all of the encouragement and organization support, barriers remain to clinical trial enrollment. These include lack of interest by oncologists and patients, limited access to trials, excessive bureaucratic demands, inadequate financial support, and the difficulty to take the time to do the hard work that is necessary.

Though direct revenue is generally considered inadequate, indirect revenue may increase by reducing patient outmigration from the hospital and physician practice, increasing referrals from community physicians and clinics and spin-off laboratory and imaging revenues.

FUNDING

An ASCO survey by Baer and colleagues[9] indicated a trend toward decreasing participation in NCI-supported clinical trials and an increase in industry-sponsored trials. One of the factors cited was that the NCI reimbursed less than 50% of actual costs incurred, a problem that continues in our current program. Booth and colleagues[10] reported a significant increase in for-profit or mixed sponsorship clinical trials. They reviewed 321 randomized clinical trials covering breast, colorectal, and non–small cell lung cancer published from 1975 to 2004. There was a significant increase from 4% to 57% of for-profit or mixed sponsorship studies over that time. During that same period, government funded randomized clinical trials decreased from 60% (28 of 47) to 31% (51 of 167).

More recent randomized clinical trials also seem to be larger and include more trial centers. Peppercorn and colleagues[11] examined breast cancer trials published in 1993, 1998, and 2003. The authors found the pharmaceutical trials to be more directed to advanced stage or likely to report a single-arm nonrandomized design. These pharmaceutical trials were also not likely to do as many head-to-head drug studies and more likely to report positive results.

Reimbursement from industry-sponsored trials is significantly better than that from cooperative groups. This allows physician and hospital trial programs to perhaps be at least budget neutral. But this is an area of potential conflict of interest, however, and has many implications in the conduct and success of clinical trials and research in general. It has been addressed in a series of articles published in the New England Journal of Medicine from 2000 through 2009.[12–15] The impact of academic and industry relationship on clinical trials is an interesting issue that will not be further addressed in this article. In spite of these changes and pressures, the percentage of clinical trials at Florida Hospital Cancer Institute (FHCI) sponsored by industry has remained approximately 33% since 1995. The clinical trials available to us are constantly reviewed, and we are currently pursuing development and participation in the Community Clinical Oncology Program. To do so certainly requires a strong commitment by the medical staff and significant administrative support, given the reimbursement issues in today's financial climate.

FLORIDA HOSPITAL CANCER INSTITUTE

The Florida Hospital in Orlando was founded in 1908 and has grown into a 1000-bed facility today. The most significant growth has been within the last 10 to 15 years when there has been increase in bed capacity and expansion of multiple programs. Six other hospitals have been incorporated into a system covering 3 counties. The original facility functions as the main or tertiary center for the system.

The FHCI was initiated in 1985, and the oncology clinical research program was started in 1989. From 1989 to 1991, there was only one nurse covering 11 medical oncologists and support staff varied between 1 and 2 people. Since then the number of staff has increased dramatically. This has been a function of sheer patient volume and clinical trial requirements for data collection for the life of the patient. Increasing patient survival has thus resulted in increasing staffing needs. There are now 16 nurses, 3 regulatory staff, 3 data managers, 1 office manager, and more than

28 physicians involved in the clinical trials program. This research team works with the participating physicians and provides staff and family education, implements protocols, organizes the consenting process, helps monitor test results, and collects and organizes data.

The original and continued structure of the program is as a hospital-based program with a centralized staff performing eligibility evaluation, trial oversight, and data management. All trial reimbursement comes to the central clinical trials office and helps to offset the costs of the clinical trials nurses and support staff. None of the reimbursement goes to the participating physicians. As previously noted, the actual costs of the trials can be substantially greater than the sponsor reimbursement, particularly from the NCI. This strongly suggests how critical it is to have FHCI administrative support, understanding the importance of the trials program in spite of its financial costs.

As this program began, we became affiliated with the Duke Oncology Consortium through which we could participate in cooperative trials. Over the years we have continued to expand our affiliations to include the Sarah Cannon Group in Nashville, the Texas Offender Reentry Initiative (TORI) program from University of California, LA, and the International Bone Marrow Transplant Registry.

Having a broad base of clinical trials available allows potential inclusion of many more patients. As the volume of patients has increased so has the number of nurses required to do these initial consults and evaluations. We now have 16 nurses who are responsible for these evaluations that take place at multiple sites in our system.

Though the number of trials offered per year has remained relatively stable, the number of consults per year has grown dramatically. This increase is also reflected in the number of patients enrolled on clinical trials per year. **Table 1** shows the number of trials available, consults, and clinical trial enrollment over intervals of 5 years from 1993 through 1997 and 1998 through 2002. **Table 1** also reflects the most recent data collected over a 7-year period from 2003 through 2009. The number of consults and subsequent patients enrolled had a dramatic increase as of approximately 1998, and this increase has been maintained.

It is believed that the increase in consults is directly related to the expansion of the number of tumor site–specific multidisciplinary tumor boards. In 1987, there was only 1 adult tumor board that allowed presentation of any tumor site the case presenter or moderator desired. The conference was held weekly, and typically 4 patients would be presented. Initially, the conference was more of the fascinating, interesting cases format with review of the literature and a more formal discussion. At present, cases are presented predominantly for discussion of patient management issues, review of treatment guidelines, and relevant literature. As seen in **Table 2**, the number of tumor boards dedicated to a specific tumor site has increased, particularly since 2000. **Table 2** shows the year the site-specific tumor boards were established at the FHCI. One can see a corresponding increase in consults and patient accrual in **Table 1**.

Table 1 Trials, consults, and enrollment			
Years	1994–1997	1998–2002	2003–2009
Number Trials/y	43	45	54
Number Consults/y	361	1435	1718
Number Patients Enrolled/y	69	163	106

Table 2
Tumor boards at FHCI

Year	Tumor Board	Videoconference	Host Site
1987	Adult multidisciplinary	2008	Orlando
1993	GYN oncology	—	Orlando
1996	Bone marrow	—	Orlando
1997	Pediatric oncology	—	Orlando
2000	Breast cancer	2009	Orlando
2002	Adult multidisciplinary	—	Altamonte
2004	Adult multidisciplinary	—	Celebration
2005	Head and neck	—	Winter Park
2008	Urology	2009	Celebration
2008	Adult multidisciplinary	—	East Orlando
2009	Colorectal	2009	Orlando
2010	Urology	2009	Orlando

Our experience has been observed by others. A study done by Kuroki and colleagues[16] from the Women and Infants Hospital in Rhode Island analyzed 1213 cases involving 916 women. They found that patients identified by the tumor board were 2.5 times more likely to enroll in a clinical trial. Vetto and colleagues[17] reported their experience at the Portland Veterans Affairs Medical Center in Portland, Oregon in 1996. Changing from "interesting" or "unusual" cases to a working conference resulted in a significant increase in the number of registered cases being presented. Most of the physicians surveyed in that study believed the working format was better for patient care and facilitated protocol enrollment. The experience at FHCI reflects those findings and supports their conclusions. Physicians have been much more willing and eager to present their patients.

As the FHCI system has grown, we have been able to provide videoconferencing to a number of our satellite campuses. As seen in **Table 2**, the originating site may actually be at one of the satellite campuses. The teleconference includes imaging, pathology, and physician discussion, with ability to communicate amongst the multiple sites. In 2009, there were a total of 448 patients presented at the various tumor boards held that year. At each of the tumor board presentations there are clinical trials nurses present to assist with clinical trial options and potential eligibility. By having all of the information immediately available and having a multidisciplinary group of physicians participating, it is much easier to assess and accrue patients for clinical trials. Using breast cancer as an example, from 1989 through 1999 there was an average of 12.5 patients per year on a breast cancer clinical trial. In the year 2000, the breast cancer–dedicated tumor conference was begun and initially met monthly but now meets up to 3 times a month. From 2000 through the first 6 months of 2010, there is now an average of 29.1 patients per year on a breast cancer clinical trial.

PATIENT CARE NAVIGATORS

The first patient navigation program was established by Dr Harold Freeman at Harlem Hospital Center in New York City. In 2003, there were more than 200 cancer programs providing navigation services designed to provide assistance for patients and families in overcoming system barriers and facilitate timely care.[18] The cancer care coordinator program at the FHCI was initiated in 2000. Services provided by our coordinators include scheduling consultations with the multidisciplinary physician team, expedite scheduling of tests and procedures, provide patient and family education, and facilitate access to clinical trials and patient/caregiver support programs. A breast cancer care coordinator position was established along with the start of the breast cancer site-specific tumor board the same year. As already noted earlier, there has been over a doubling of patients accrued to breast cancer clinical trials since the inception of the care coordinator and site-specific tumor board program.

Along with the increasing number of tumor board sites, there has been a progressive increase in the number of care coordinators. Since the first breast care coordinator started, there have been 3 additional coordinators assigned to that program. In addition, our thoracic cancer program also has a total of 3 coordinators, whereas the head and neck program, urology program, brain spine program, and gastrointestinal program each has 1 coordinator. By having early contact with a potentially large number of patients, each coordinator can direct the patient to the appropriate team of specialists. As part of the education process, general information about clinical trials can be given to patients to help them understand the trials' hopeful benefits.

THE FUTURE

The current status of clinical trial development and execution has recently been brought into question. The Institute of Medicine has indicated there needs to be a more efficient response to emerging scientific advances, improving speed and efficiency of clinical trials, improving selection and completion of clinical trials, and the fostering of expanded participation of patients and physicians.[19] By having the needed infrastructure in place for a growing clinical trials program, we believe we will be prepared to meet these challenges. Hospital administrative support, a strong clinical research staff, site-specific tumor boards, and dedicated care coordinators will help facilitate and expedite patient care and clinical trial accrual.

REFERENCES

1. Veronisi U, Bonadonna G, Valagussa P. Lessons from the initial adjuvant cyclophosphamide, methotrexate, and fluorouracil studies in operable breast cancer. J Clin Oncol 2008;26:342–4.
2. Avent R, Dillman R. Cancer clinical trials in the community setting: a 20 year retrospective. Cancer Biother 1995;10:95–113.
3. Fleming I. Barriers to clinical trials. Part I: reimbursement problems. Cancer 1994; 74:2662–5.
4. Cobau C. Clinical trials in the community: the community clinical oncology program experience. Cancer 1994;74:2694–700.
5. Wilke L, Ballman K, McCall L, et al. Adherance to the National Quality Forum (NQF) breast cancer measures within cancer clinical trials: a review from ACOSOG Z0010. Ann Surg Oncol 2010;17:1989–94.
6. Lamont E, Landrum M, Keating N, et al. Differences in clinical trial patient attributes and outcomes according to enrollment setting. J Clin Oncol 2009;28: 215–21.
7. Burstein H. Do clinical trials belong in clinical guidelines? J Natl Compr Canc Netw 2009;7:489.
8. American College of Surgeons, Commission on Cancer, Cancer Program Standards. 2009 Revised Edition. p. 63–7. Available at: http://www.facs.org/cancer/coc/cocprogramstandards.pdf. Accessed July 5, 2010.

9. Baer A, Kelly C, Bruinooge S, et al. Challenges to National Cancer Institute-supported cooperative group clinical trials participation: an ASCO survey of cooperative group sites. J Oncol Pract 2010;6:114–9.
10. Booth C, Cescon D, Wang L, et al. Evolution of the randomized controlled trial in oncology over three decades. J Clin Oncol 2008;26:5458–64.
11. Peppercorn J, Blood E, Winer E, et al. Association between pharmaceutical involvement and outcomes in breast cancer clinical trials. Cancer 2007;109: 1239–46.
12. McCrary S, Anderson C, Jakovljevic J, et al. A national survey of policies on disclosure of conflicts of interest in biomedical research. N Engl J Med 2000; 343:1621–6.
13. Blumenthal D. Academic-industrial relationships in the life sciences. N Engl J Med 2003;349:2452–9.
14. Stossel T. Regulating academic-industrial research relationships-solving problems or stifling progress? N Engl J Med 2005;353:1060–5.
15. Weinfurt K, Hall M, King N, et al. Disclosure of financial relationships to participants in clinical research. N Engl J Med 2009;361:916–21.
16. Kuroki L, Stuckey A, Hirway P, et al. Addressing clinical trials: can the multidisciplinary tumor board improve participation? A study from an academic women's cancer program. Gynecol Oncol 2010;116:295–300.
17. Vetto J, Richert-Boe K, Desler M, et al. Tumor board formats: "fascinating case" versus "working conference". J Cancer Educ 1996;11:84–8.
18. Varner A, Murph P. Cancer patient navigation: where do we go from here? Oncol Issues 2010;25(3):50–3.
19. Institute of Medicine Report. National cancer clinical trials system for the 21st century: reinvigorating the NCI cooperative group program. April 2010.

Hepatic Tumor Ablation: Application in a Community Hospital Setting

Kwan N. Lau, MD, Ryan Z. Swan, MD, David Sindram, MD, PhD, John B. Martinie, MD, David A. Iannitti, MD*

KEYWORDS

• Liver cancer • Microwave • Ablation • Radiofrequency

Primary liver tumors are a common clinical problem with a steadily increasing incidence in the United States and worldwide. The estimated death rate from primary liver and intrahepatic bile duct tumors has increased in both men and women in the United States in 2010,[1] and the incidence of liver tumors is much higher if other malignancies that routinely metastasize to the liver are taken into account. Whether primary liver cancer or metastatic disease, if left untreated, the prognosis is dismal for these patients. Resection has historically been considered the gold standard treatment for liver lesions; however, the current treatment options have been expanded to include a wide array of liver-directed therapies.[2–4] Today, commonly used liver-directed therapies include transarterial chemoembolization (TACE), selective internal radiation therapy (SIRT), and ablative therapy. All these treatment modalities can provide disease control depending on the cause of tumor. Among these different liver-directed therapy options, only ablative therapy can cause direct destruction of the targeted tissue. The commercially available modalities readily accessible to surgeons in the United States today are all based on thermoablative technology: cryosurgical therapy, monopolar radiofrequency ablation (RFA), and microwave ablation (MWA). All the 3 modalities can achieve tumor destruction; however, each modality carries distinct physical properties. Physicians should familiarize themselves with each technology to maximize its efficacy for clinical application. This article examines the various ablative technologies and their application, as well as how these procedures can be performed safely and with optimal outcomes, in a community cancer center.

Hepato-Pancreato-Biliary Surgery, Department of General Surgery, Carolinas Medical Center, 1025 Morehead Medical Plaza Drive, Suite 300, Charlotte, NC 28204, USA
* Corresponding author.
E-mail address: david.iannitti@carolinashealthcare.org

Surg Oncol Clin N Am 20 (2011) 455–466
doi:10.1016/j.soc.2011.01.003
1055-3207/11/$ – see front matter © 2011 Elsevier Inc. All rights reserved.

BASIC PRINCIPLES OF THERMOABLATIVE TECHNOLOGY

Human cells are susceptible to thermal injury, and permanent cell damage is caused at extreme temperatures ($<-100°C$ or $>50°C$). Cell exposure to temperatures greater than $50°C$, even for as short as 4 to 6 minutes, results in protein denaturation that causes irreversible cell death.[5] The formation of intracellular ice crystals, when cells are subjected to temperatures less than $-40°C$, causes lethal cell damage by microcirculatory failure[6] and cellular necrosis.[7] This article discusses the interaction of each therapy with local tissue factors and how this interaction plays a role in determining the final ablative zone.

CRYOSURGICAL THERAPY

The application of cryosurgical ablation began in the 1960s, and the cryogens commonly used were nitrous oxide, liquid nitrogen, and argon. The general setup of cryosurgical devices use a segmental insulated probe through which the cryogen is delivered, causing rapid expansion of the cryogenic gas, with rapid cooling to temperatures approaching $-100°C$ in a few seconds. The common cryogens used for hepatic ablation are liquid nitrogen and argon, with the latter using a smaller-size probe and a more-rapid freeze cycle. The small size of its applicator permits percutaneous use. The thawing of the resulting ice ball is facilitated by instillation of helium gas. It is recommended that a rapid freeze, followed by a slow thaw, then repeat freeze-thaw cycles be used for maximal effect. The advantage of cryosurgery is its ability to be visualized on computed tomography (CT) and magnetic resonance imaging (MRI) because of ice ball formation. A 3-cm ice ball can be generated through a single applicator, and larger areas of freezing can be achieved by overlapping multiple applicators. A niche application of cryosurgical ablation is for lesions located adjacent to a major vessel because the heating effect of flowing blood is protective to the vessel.[6,8]

MONOPOLAR RFA

The most widely used thermoablative technology worldwide is monopolar RFA, which uses an electrosurgical device operating at 200 to 1200 kHz on the electromagnetic spectrum. It is estimated that 90% of all ablations performed in the United States are monopolar RFAs. Monopolar RFA requires a closed circuit to function, which means grounding pads (active electrodes) must be applied to the patient, similar to electrosurgery. Alternating current is passed between the RFA electrode and the grounding pad. The rapidly oscillating current passing between the electrode and the grounding pad causes agitation of intracellular ions and leads to frictional heat formation. The heat energy generated leads to coagulative necrosis by conduction and is concentrated around the electrode because of higher current density secondary to its smaller surface area.[9]

The clinical effects of RFA can be heavily influenced by the location of the lesion because current follows the path of least electrical resistance. This property can create a clinical problem when the electrode is in close proximity to a large blood vessel because blood vessels have lower impedance than the surrounding tissue. Current can be diverted away from the target area under these conditions, which can lead to smaller or more irregular ablation zones than anticipated. This phenomenon is known as electrical sink, a concept similar to thermal sink, in which heat is being shunted away by the flowing blood.[10]

The rapid increase in tissue temperature around the RFA electrode can limit the efficacy of RFA because of tissue desiccation and charring. During RFA, it is imperative to maintain the target tissue temperature at less than 100°C to prevent tissue vaporization and carbonization, which increases the impedance significantly and hinders current flow.[11] The commercially available systems optimize power output through an impedance-based or output-based system. These improvements in design for RFA allow an ablation diameter up to 4 to 5 cm with multiple electrodes used in combination; however, the local tissue effects discussed earlier may still decrease or alter the final ablative volume. Other improvements to RFA include the use of multiprong electrodes to allow larger current deposition and more predictable heating,[12] as well as coupling of the electrodes to temperature or impedance sensors to allow real-time feedback and adjustment of energy output based on a preset algorithm to achieve effective ablation. Saline infusion within the shaft of the electrode can reduce the tissue temperature for a better electrode-tissue interface,[13] and pulsed delivery of radiofrequency energy has also been developed to maximize current deposition.[14] The next generation of radiofrequency technology is the development of bipolar RFA, and it is currently being used in selected centers in the United States. The deployment of 2 electrodes completes the circuit required; therefore, no grounding pad is necessary for bipolar RFA. However, reports on the clinical results for bipolar RFA are currently lacking.

MWA

MWA also uses radiofrequency energy, but it operates at a much higher frequency (900 MHz–10 GHz) than RFA. The energy deposition for MWA is also completely different from that for RFA. The MWA antenna broadcasts nonionizing radiation to achieve tissue destruction, and a grounding pad is not necessary because there is no flow of current. Heat generation by MWA is effected by water molecules, which orient themselves within the applied electromagnetic field. The dipole characteristic of water molecules causes them to orient toward the polarity of the rapidly changing electromagnetic field. This rapid alternation in polarity generates heat energy via vibration in a process termed dielectric hysteresis.[15]

The distinct characteristic of MWA is its ability to homogeneously broadcast energy throughout its near field, which is largely defined by the microwave frequency and antenna configuration. All tissues in this zone are heated homogenously without being influenced by local tissue factors such as close proximity to blood vessels. These properties distinguish MWA from RFA and render MWA a more attractive option for hepatic ablation. However, in tissue that does not fall within the volume of the near field of microwave, the heating is conductive (as in RFA), and the tissue is hence susceptible to thermal sink. Given the superior physical properties and ease of use, microwave technology will replace monopolar RFA in the treatment of liver tumors.[16]

Three microwave frequencies have been approved for clinical use in the United States: 915 MHz, 2.45 GHz, and 9.2 GHz. Only the manufacturers of the 915-MHz (Valleylab, Boulder, CO, USA) and 2.45-GHz (Acculis Ltd, Microsulis Medical Ltd, Denmead, UK) systems have US Food and Drug Administration (FDA)-approved commercially available systems for liver tumor ablation, and the authors use both systems in their institution. The 915-MHz system uses a solid-state amplifier to generate microwave energy, whereas the 2.45-GHz system uses a magnetron. Both systems have proved to be effective in the authors' experience, as each system has its distinct properties and advantages. The difference in frequency theoretically permits deeper tissue penetration with the 915-MHz system, whereas the 2.45-GHz system is capable of higher energy deposition within the electromagnetic field given a similar wattage.

The selection of system depends on the number of lesions and their location. The 915-MHz system uses a smaller antenna (13 gauge), which allows percutaneous application. It is often used in a clustered triple antenna formation to treat larger (>3-cm diameter) lesions, with the customary settings at 45 W for 10 minutes powered by 3 different 915-MHz generators. The 2.45-GHz system has a larger size (5-mm diameter) antenna and can produce comparable ablative sizes with 100 W over a 5-minute setting with 1 antenna alone. A smaller (1.8 mm) percutaneous antenna for the 2.45-GHz system has recently been approved by the FDA, which may expand its clinical usage.

EXPERIMENTAL MODALITIES

High-intensity focused ultrasonography (HIFU) and irreversible electroporation (IRE) are experimental modalities on the horizon for hepatic ablation that are showing some promise. The arrival of these new technologies may supplement current technology and help define niche application for each modality in treating liver tumors.

HIFU

The attractive feature of HIFU is its ability to achieve coagulative necrosis without using an invasive applicator. The probe of HIFU can focus an ultrasound beam to an intensity of 100 to 10,000 W/cm^2 and increase its peak compression and rarefaction pressure up to 30 and 100 MPa, respectively. Comparatively, diagnostic ultrasonography uses only 0.1 to 100 mW/cm^2 or compression and rarefaction pressures of 0.001 to 0.003 MPa, depending on the mode of imaging. The acoustic energy is then converted to heat energy within the tissue, and coagulative necrosis is achieved within a focal region. The energy distribution of HIFU is confined to within 1 mm in diameter. The clinical advantage of such a precise application is that the effect of undesired thermal spread can be limited, which is often the undesired effect of other thermoablative technologies. HIFU was first developed to treat other areas of the body, such as the eye, prostate, and kidney. Initial investigation of HIFU in ablating liver lesions has shown some promising results. A randomized trial has compared TACE alone with TACE and HIFU for the treatment of hepatocellular cancer. The HIFU-TACE group demonstrated a survival benefit of 6 months over the TACE-alone group.[17] Research is ongoing to define its role in treating hepatic tumors.

Irreversible Electroporation

Irreversible electroporation (IRE) is a distinct class of ablative therapy because it does not cause tissue necrosis by a thermal means. IRE works by delivering a high-voltage differential (1000–3000 V) across 1 cm for the duration of milliseconds to microseconds, inducing nanodefects on the cell membrane.[18,19] The permanent defects disrupt cell homeostasis, and cell death ensues.[20] The effect of IRE is different among different tissue types. Whereas IRE spares bile ducts and blood vessels, its primary effect is on the liver parenchymal cells. There are animal studies to support IRE as an ablative option,[21,22] but clinical trials are currently lacking. Recently, a commercially available machine has been introduced in the United States, which makes IRE an exciting new option for liver tumor ablation.

OUTCOME FOR ABLATIVE THERAPIES
Hepatocellular Carcinoma

Hepatocellular carcinoma (HCC) poses a significant clinical problem worldwide and in the United States because of its tumor biology and increasing incidence. HCC is the third leading cause of cancer death worldwide, and its incidence is steadily increasing in the United States.[1,23] It is believed that viral hepatitis, especially hepatitis C, along with obesity and alcohol abuse, contributes significantly to the development of cirrhosis in the United States, which is the leading risk factor for developing HCC.

The clinical spectrum of HCC is diverse, and no staging scheme has been successful in accurately describing all the scenarios. However, HCC can usually be classified into local or regional disease and intrahepatic or extrahepatic metastases while factoring in patients' underlying hepatic function.[24] Local disease usually refers to a single small lesion, and the treatment intent is curative. The goal would be to remove the tumor, either by resection or by ablation. However, if patients have advanced disease, the focus should be on disease control, and patients can benefit from some combinations of liver-directed therapy.

There are 3 main treatment strategies for HCC depending on the clinical stage, each of which is potentially curative: resectional therapy (RT), orthotopic liver transplant (OLT), and ablative therapy. Historically, RT and OLT have the best 5-year survival rate, with up to a reported rate of 70%.[25] However, only select patients are candidates for RT, and many patients cannot undergo resection because of underlying parenchymal disease with inadequate hepatic reserve, multiple tumors, unfavorable tumor location, and/or other prohibitive medical comorbidities. Patients who are candidates for RT usually have a small tumor and normal liver function, and this is the recommended treatment option by the European Association for the Study of the Liver and the American Association for the Study of Liver Diseases.[26–28] The recurrence rate for RT at 5 years, however, can reach as high as 70%,[29,30] especially for patients who have tumors larger than 5 cm, 3 or more tumors, vascular invasion, and/or a narrow resection margin.

There are strict selection criteria for OLT, the most widely used being the Milan criteria. These patients have either a single HCC of up to 5 cm or up to 3 tumors, with none more than 3 cm.[31] OLT has the advantage of treating both the HCC and the underlying liver disease; however, the time on the wait list can be variable, and up to 10% to 30% drop out rates have been reported.[29] Effort has been made to allocate additional MELD (model of end stage liver disease) score points in hopes of shortening the waiting period for patients with HCC. These additional MELD points are maintained following ablation of HCC, whereas they are lost following resection, making ablation the preferred treatment modality for lesions smaller than 5 cm as a bridge to transplant. However, the scarcity of suitable organs remains a major hurdle for the widespread implementation of OLT as a treatment option.

Ablation therapy has been extensively studied in the treatment of HCC and demonstrated to provide adequate locoregional disease control in patients with small-volume disease alone. Patients who cannot undergo resection or who are poor surgical candidates can also benefit from ablative therapy as one of the components of liver-directed therapy for disease control, which commonly entails selective internal radiation therapy,[32] TACE,[33] or portal vein embolization.

Ablative therapy for HCC has evolved from cryosurgical therapy and monopolar RFA to now include MWA. The series confirming the role of cryosurgical ablation for HCC mostly involve open intraoperative application in the 1990s, and good results were reported with tumors less than 5 cm in diameter.[34,35] The 1-, 3-, and 5-year survival rates of patients with tumors smaller than 5 cm were reported as 97%, 77%, and 55%, respectively, in a series of 235 patients.[35] However, for patients with tumors larger than 5 cm, the 5-year survival rate was only 25%. Percutaneous application of cryosurgical ablation for treating HCC is not widely reported. Patients with a tumor burden replacing more than 40% of the liver content are poor candidates for cryotherapy. One devastating complication for cryosurgical therapy is cryoshock, which entails severe coagulopathy and multiorgan failure.[36,37] The incidence of cryoshock is estimated at 1%, but it carries a 28% reported mortality. Cracking of the ice ball (<25%), hemorrhage (<13%), bile fistula/biloma (<10%), abscess (0%–9%), pleural effusion (4%–18%), and death (0%–8%) are other observed complications.[38] Despite the proven clinical value of cryosurgical therapy, it has been replaced by thermoablative therapy (monopolar RFA and MWA), because of their ease of use, better safety profile, and shorter application time.

The most studied modality in ablative therapy for HCC is monopolar RFA, which accounts for 90% of all liver ablation worldwide.[39] The 3 commercially available systems (AngioDynamics, Latham, NY, USA; Boston Scientific, Natick, MA, USA; and Valleylab) have all been shown to be equally effective for HCC up to 3 cm.[13] Excellent results have been reported for treating HCC with RFA for different tumor sizes: less than 3 cm, 3 to 5 cm, and greater than 5 cm.[40–43] There have been reports suggesting that RFA should be the treatment of choice for patients with small HCC (<2 cm), including those who have Child class A cirrhosis.[43] In one retrospective study of 218 patients, the local recurrence rate was 2.8% and complication rate was 1.8%. There have been randomized trials suggesting that survival rates for patients with small HCC were similar when treated with RT or RFA.[41,42] However, the recurrence rate of RFA could be as high as 14.9% as reported in a large meta-analysis of 2369 cases of HCC ablation.[44] One of the challenges for treating small HCC by RFA is the difficulty in targeting the small lesion, especially via the percutaneous route. Another concern is that RFA has an inferior physical profile (compared with MWA, as discussed earlier), which renders incomplete ablation possible. The advancement of modern ablative technology and the improvement in lesion targeting would improve the local recurrence rate.

The treatment of HCC using MWA is still in its early stage in the United States, but extensive experience using MWA in Asia and Europe has been reported with good results.[45–47] The FDA first approved the clinical application of MWA in 2008 following clinical trials that confirmed the efficacy of MWA in producing complete tumor destruction. These findings were confirmed by immunohistochemical analysis in the ablation zone in all 11 patients who underwent hepatoma ablation followed by resection, with an average reported ablation diameter of 5.5 cm.[48] A subsequent phase 2 trial enrolled 87 patients, of which 23 had HCC, and at a mean follow-up of 19 months, 47% of patients were alive without evidence of disease.[49] The reported local recurrence was 2.3%. A similar local recurrence rate (2%) was observed in another series.[50] MWA also demonstrated a promising survival rate: 1-, 3-, and 5-year survival rates were reported as 97%, 81%, and 43%, respectively.[51] Other series have examined the role of MWA in larger lesions, and a 44% 3-year survival rate has been reported in a series of 69 patients with HCC up to 4 cm in diameter.[52]

Colorectal Liver Metastases

Each year, more than 140,000 cases of colorectal cancer are diagnosed in the United States, and there are 50,000 cancer deaths related to colorectal cancer yearly.[23] It is the third leading cancer-related cause of death, and many patients (up to two-thirds) develop metastases, most commonly to the liver.

The treatment of colorectal liver metastases (CRLM) is evolving, and the choice of treatments depends on multiple factors, including tumor burden, tumor location, number of lesions, and tumor responsiveness to chemotherapeutic agents. Ideally, patients who are amenable to resection should receive RT, but only 10% to 25% of patients are candidates for RT.[53] The advancement in neoadjuvant chemotherapeutic agents has demonstrated that up to 38% of patients can potentially be down staged and become candidates for RT.[54] The survival rate for patients undergoing hepatic resection has improved significantly compared with earlier studies, with reported 5- and 10-year survival rates as high as 71% and 60%, respectively.[55] Treatment strategies focused on liver-directed therapy have been developed to provide alterative treatments for disease control. Ablative therapy, in conjunction with TACE and SIRT, has significantly improved the survival of these patients, who otherwise would have a 5-year survival rate of 0% to 1% if left untreated.[56,57]

There are case series reporting the treatment of CRLM with cryosurgical and ethanol ablation with good results,[58,59] but the newer modalities, RFA and MWA, have largely made ethanol and cryosurgical ablation an historical interest only. As with HCC, RFA is the most studied modality for treating CRLM, with excellent 1-, 2-, and 3-year survival rates reported as 87%, 77%, and 50%, respectively.[40] Multiple other series have confirmed the role of RFA as an effective treatment for CRLM.[60–62] Long-term survival meta-analysis data for RFA have shown that percutaneous application can lead to lower rates of local disease control and an increased risk of tumor tracking.[44] This study also suggested that surgical RFA is an effective treatment for CRLM less than 3 cm, with results comparable with RT. It is believed that the high recurrence rate for RFA may be intrinsic to its physical limitation, especially if perivascular lesions are treated.[10] The addition of MWA, along with image guidance for lesion targeting, should minimize the risks of local recurrence and improve overall survival.

Clinical studies have emerged in the literature validating MWA as an effective treatment for CRLM.[48,63,64] The local recurrence and 3-year survival rates reported are encouraging, and a small randomized controlled trial (n = 30) has demonstrated that MWA and RT have similar overall survival rates.[48,64] Patient management for CRLM should involve a multidisciplinary approach to determine the best treatment plan. Generally, a cytoreductive strategy is advocated if the morbidity and mortality risks of the treatment are low. However, the underlying biology of CRLM is different for each patient, and treatment should be tailored individually. Aggressive tumor biology of CRLM has been defined, and features such as positive margins, extrahepatic disease, node-positive primary, disease-free interval from primary to metastasis of less than 12 months, more than 1 hepatic tumor, largest hepatic tumor greater than 5 cm, and carcinoembryonic antigen level greater than 200 ng/mL are associated with a poor outcome with RT.[65] However, even for patients with extrahepatic disease, adequate locoregional disease control can still improve outcomes.[66] MWA provides an effective option for treating CRLM, as it has a lower complication profile than resection and is capable of complete tumor destruction.

Neuroendocrine Tumors and Metastasis from Other Primary Tumors

Neuroendocrine tumors and other primary cancers, such as breast carcinoma and genitourinary tumors that metastasize to the liver, are traditionally evaluated for hepatic resection. Improved survival has been reported in selected patients who undergo RT for noncolorectal/nonneuroendocrine metastases.[67] In regards to neuroendocrine metastases, not unlike HCC and CRLM, 90% of these patients are not candidates for hepatic resection, and many of them remain symptomatic from local and endocrine effect. Curative and palliative resections are possible only in 20% to 25% of these patients, but these resections can relieve symptoms for more than 2 years in 90% of the patients. Five-year survival is prolonged to 40% to 85%, although metastases recur or progress in almost all patients.[68] RFA has been used for endocrine symptom palliation, and 70% to 90% of patients have a good effect for 2 years. Other liver-directed therapies, such as chemoembolization and embolization, have been used to treat patients not amenable to surgical treatment (RT and RFA), with an observed 50% tumor burden reduction and 60% 5-year survival rates.[68]

ESSENTIAL COMPONENTS OF A LIVER ABLATION PROGRAM

Liver ablation is an effective treatment for primary and metastatic hepatic tumors, as discussed earlier in this article. Providing ablative therapy to the liver requires significant resources from the hospital, coordination between different departments, and surgical expertise in hepatobiliary surgery. Unlike pancreatic surgery, there is currently no literature outlining the specific hospital setting in which ablative therapy should be delivered, and there is no surgeon or hospital annual volume recommendation. Nevertheless, ablation therapy for liver tumors does require significant training and should be used in the greater context of a liver-directed therapy program. The following paragraphs detail the essential components necessary for the development of a successful ablative program.

Carolinas Medical Center, a 1000-bed academic medical center located in Charlotte, North Carolina, is the flagship hospital of the Carolinas Healthcare System.[69] The Hepato-Pancreato-Biliary (HPB) Program was established in 2006 in response to increasing demand and currently serves the population of central and western North Carolina. Clinically, there are 3 dedicated staff HPB consultants, all of whom are fellowship-trained and familiar with the various ablative techniques. The service provides full-time coverage for all HPB-related diseases and is composed of HPB surgeons, surgical fellows/residents, and physician extenders.

Surgeons who perform ablative therapy should receive the appropriate training, ideally including didactic and practice sessions, to familiarize themselves with the system they are using, as there are significant and potentially dangerous differences between the various forms of ablative technology. In addition to familiarity with the ablation instrumentation, successful ablation requires expertise in intraoperative ultrasonography (open and laparoscopic), and the surgeon must know how to interpret the images to accurately target the lesion. The commercial availability of RFA and MWA has expanded the pool of practitioners who are able to deliver liver ablative therapy and makes it feasible to perform these procedures outside the traditional regional tertiary referral center. However, it cannot be overstated that ablative therapy is only one of the options in the much broader scope of treating hepatic malignancies. This total care approach requires additional resources be in place to enact the best treatment plan for patients.

It is imperative that patients be discussed in a multidisciplinary approach, and involvement of medical and radiation oncology early on is crucial in determining the timing of the ablation and the coordination of additional chemotherapy and/or radiation therapy for an optimal outcome. If the best treatment for a patient is resection or transplant, the patient needs to be seen by or referred to the corresponding service, and the treatment cannot be biased toward ablation if these other options are not available.

During the ablation procedure, familiarity of the anesthesia team with treating patients with liver disease is a crucial part of ensuring a good postablation outcome and is especially important for volume management in cirrhotic patients. The operating room staff must be familiar with the setup of the ablation equipment, and the surgeons should know the basics of how to operate and troubleshoot the system. Ideally, the surgeon should be capable of performing hepatic surgery because rare but severe complications can occur with hepatic ablation. Full-time coverage by board-certified intensivists and the assistance of experienced hepatologists are crucial to optimize patients' postoperative care, especially in patients with advanced liver disease.

Cross-sectional imaging, such as triphasic liver CT scan and MRI, are needed to evaluate the result of ablative therapy, and radiologists with expertise in reading post-ablation imaging are essential for monitoring recurrence. At present, all patients undergoing ablation at Carolinas Medical Center receive imaging 1 month postoperatively to rule out incomplete ablation, then every 4 months for 2 years and every 6 months thereafter.

Another valuable resource from the radiology department is the availability of interventional radiologists who can provide periablative support such as percutaneous biopsy, arterial embolization, or drainage procedures. Also, they can provide patients with the options of receiving other liver-directed therapies such as TACE and SIRT as part of a comprehensive treatment plan.

SUMMARY

Liver ablation can be performed safely in a tertiary care community cancer center, provided that the appropriate surgeon training and substantial hospital support structure are in place. A multimodal strategy of liver-directed and systemic therapy should be available to provide the full range of treatment options for primary and metastatic hepatic tumors, of which ablative therapy is an essential component.

REFERENCES

1. Jemal A, Siegel R, Xu J, et al. Cancer statistics, 2010. CA Cancer J Clin 2010; 60(5):277–300.
2. Llovet JM, Real MI, Montana X, et al. Arterial embolisation or chemoembolisation versus symptomatic treatment in patients with unresectable hepatocellular carcinoma: a randomised controlled trial. Lancet 2002;359(9319):1734–9.
3. Bruix J, Llovet JM. Prognostic prediction and treatment strategy in hepatocellular carcinoma. Hepatology 2002;35(3):519–24.
4. Tsuzuki T, Sugioka A, Ueda M, et al. Hepatic resection for hepatocellular carcinoma. Surgery 1990;107(5):511–20.
5. Larson TR, Bostwick DG, Corica A. Temperature-correlated histopathologic changes following microwave thermoablation of obstructive tissue in patients with benign prostatic hyperplasia. Urology 1996;47(4):463–9.
6. Mascarenhas BA, Ravikumar TS. Experimental basis for hepatic cryotherapy. Semin Surg Oncol 1998;14(2):110–5.
7. McCarty TM, Kuhn JA. Cryotherapy for liver tumors. Oncology (Williston Park) 1998;12(7):979–87 [discussion: 990, 993].
8. Wong WS, Patel SC, Cruz FS, et al. Cryosurgery as a treatment for advanced stage hepatocellular carcinoma: results, complications, and alcohol ablation. Cancer 1998;82(7):1268–78.
9. Brace CL. Radiofrequency and microwave ablation of the liver, lung, kidney, and bone: what are the differences? Curr Probl Diagn Radiol 2009;38(3): 135–43.
10. Livraghi T, Goldberg SN, Lazzaroni S, et al. Hepatocellular carcinoma: radiofrequency ablation of medium and large lesions. Radiology 2000;214(3):761–8.
11. Dadd JS, Ryan TP, Platt R. Tissue impedance as a function of temperature and time. Biomed Sci Instrum 1996;32:205–14.
12. Hope WW, Arru JM, McKee JQ, et al. Evaluation of multiprobe radiofrequency technology in a porcine model. HPB (Oxford) 2007;9(5):363–7.

13. Shibata T, Maetani Y, Isoda H, et al. Radiofrequency ablation for small hepatocellular carcinoma: prospective comparison of internally cooled electrode and expandable electrode. Radiology 2006;238(1):346–53.

14. Cua IH, Lin CC, Lin CJ, et al. Treatment of hepatocellular carcinoma using internally cooled electrodes. A prospective comparison of modified automated vs. manual pulsed radiofrequency algorithms. Oncology 2007;72(Suppl 1):76–82.

15. Brace CL. Microwave ablation technology: what every user should know. Curr Probl Diagn Radiol 2009;38(2):61–7.

16. Nicholl MB, Conway CW, Xing Y, et al. Should microwave energy be preferred to radiofrequency energy for ablation of malignant liver tumors? J Interv Oncol 2010;3(1):12–6.

17. Wu F, Wang ZB, Chen WZ, et al. Advanced hepatocellular carcinoma: treatment with high-intensity focused ultrasound ablation combined with transcatheter arterial embolization. Radiology 2005;235(2):659–67.

18. Miller L, Leor J, Rubinsky B. Cancer cells ablation with irreversible electroporation. Technol Cancer Res Treat 2005;4(6):699–705.

19. Edd JF, Horowitz L, Davalos RV, et al. In vivo results of a new focal tissue ablation technique: irreversible electroporation. IEEE Trans Biomed Eng 2006;53(7):1409–15.

20. Rubinsky B. Irreversible electroporation in medicine. Technol Cancer Res Treat 2007;6(4):255–60.

21. Al-Sakere B, Andre F, Bernat C, et al. Tumor ablation with irreversible electroporation. PLoS One 2007;2(11):e1135.

22. Al-Sakere B, Bernat C, Andre F, et al. A study of the immunological response to tumor ablation with irreversible electroporation. Technol Cancer Res Treat 2007; 6(4):301–6.

23. Edwards BK, Ward E, Kohler BA, et al. Annual report to the nation on the status of cancer, 1975–2006, featuring colorectal cancer trends and impact of interventions (risk factors, screening, and treatment) to reduce future rates. Cancer 2010;116(3):544–73.

24. Sindram D, Lau KN, Martinie JB, et al. Hepatic tumor ablation. Surg Clin North Am 2010;90(4):863–76.

25. Llovet JM, Burroughs A, Bruix J. Hepatocellular carcinoma. Lancet 2003; 362(9399):1907–17.

26. Bruix J, Sherman M, Llovet JM, et al. Clinical management of hepatocellular carcinoma. Conclusions of the Barcelona-2000 EASL conference. European Association for the Study of the Liver. J Hepatol 2001;35(3):421–30.

27. Bruix J, Sherman M. Management of hepatocellular carcinoma. Hepatology 2005; 42(5):1208–36.

28. Kao JH, Chen DS. Local ablation vs. resection for the treatment of hepatocellular carcinoma. Hepatology 2006;43(2):373.

29. Llovet JM, Schwartz M, Mazzaferro V. Resection and liver transplantation for hepatocellular carcinoma. Semin Liver Dis 2005;25(2):181–200.

30. Schwartz JD, Schwartz M, Mandeli J, et al. Neoadjuvant and adjuvant therapy for resectable hepatocellular carcinoma: review of the randomised clinical trials. Lancet Oncol 2002;3(10):593–603.

31. Mazzaferro V, Regalia E, Doci R, et al. Liver transplantation for the treatment of small hepatocellular carcinomas in patients with cirrhosis. N Engl J Med 1996; 334(11):693–9.

32. Cianni R, Urigo C, Notarianni E, et al. Selective internal radiation therapy with SIR-spheres for the treatment of unresectable colorectal hepatic metastases. Cardiovasc Intervent Radiol 2009;32(6):1179–86.

33. Rathore R, Safran H, Soares G, et al. Phase I study of hepatic arterial infusion of oxaliplatin in advanced hepatocellular cancer: a brown university oncology group study. Am J Clin Oncol 2009;33(1):43–6.
34. Zhou XD, Tang ZY, Yu YQ. Ablative approach for primary liver cancer: Shanghai experience. Surg Oncol Clin N Am 1996;5(2):379–90.
35. Zhou XD, Tang ZY. Cryotherapy for primary liver cancer. Semin Surg Oncol 1998; 14(2):171–4.
36. Seifert JK, Junginger T, Morris DL. A collective review of the world literature on hepatic cryotherapy. J R Coll Surg Edinb 1998;43(3):141–54.
37. Seifert JK, Morris DL. World survey on the complications of hepatic and prostate cryotherapy. World J Surg 1999;23(2):109–13 [discussion: 113–4].
38. Kosowski K, Nowak W, Dancewicz W, et al. Cryotherapy of liver tumors. Przegl Lek 2005;62(12):1436–9 [in Polish].
39. Sutherland LM, Williams JA, Padbury RT, et al. Radiofrequency ablation of liver tumors: a systematic review. Arch Surg 2006;141(2):181–90.
40. Iannitti DA, Dupuy DE, Mayo-Smith WW, et al. Hepatic radiofrequency ablation. Arch Surg 2002;137(4):422–6 [discussion: 427].
41. Chen MS, Li JQ, Zheng Y, et al. A prospective randomized trial comparing percutaneous local ablative therapy and partial hepatectomy for small hepatocellular carcinoma. Ann Surg 2006;243(3):321–8.
42. Lu MD, Kuang M, Liang LJ, et al. Surgical resection versus percutaneous thermal ablation for early-stage hepatocellular carcinoma: a randomized clinical trial. Zhonghua Yi Xue Za Zhi 2006;86(12):801–5 [in Chinese].
43. Livraghi T, Meloni F, Di Stasi M, et al. Sustained complete response and complications rates after radiofrequency ablation of very early hepatocellular carcinoma in cirrhosis: is resection still the treatment of choice? Hepatology 2008;47(1): 82–9.
44. Mulier S, Ni Y, Jamart J, et al. Local recurrence after hepatic radiofrequency coagulation: multivariate meta-analysis and review of contributing factors. Ann Surg 2005;242(2):158–71.
45. Seki T, Tamai T, Nakagawa T, et al. Combination therapy with transcatheter arterial chemoembolization and percutaneous microwave coagulation therapy for hepatocellular carcinoma. Cancer 2000;89(6):1245–51.
46. Lu MD, Chen JW, Xie XY, et al. Hepatocellular carcinoma: US-guided percutaneous microwave coagulation therapy. Radiology 2001;221(1):167–72.
47. Shibata T, Iimuro Y, Yamamoto Y, et al. Small hepatocellular carcinoma: comparison of radio-frequency ablation and percutaneous microwave coagulation therapy. Radiology 2002;223(2):331–7.
48. Simon CJ, Dupuy DE, Iannitti DA, et al. Intraoperative triple antenna hepatic microwave ablation. AJR Am J Roentgenol 2006;187(4):W333–40.
49. Iannitti DA, Martin RC, Simon CJ, et al. Hepatic tumor ablation with clustered microwave antennae: the US phase II trial. HPB (Oxford) 2007;9(2):120–4.
50. Martin RC, Scoggins CR, McMasters KM. Safety and efficacy of microwave ablation of hepatic tumors: a prospective review of a 5-year experience. Ann Surg Oncol 2010;17(1):171–8.
51. Seki S, Sakaguchi H, Iwai S, et al. Five-year survival of patients with hepatocellular carcinoma treated with laparoscopic microwave coagulation therapy. Endoscopy 2005;37(12):1220–5.
52. Kawamoto C, Ido K, Isoda N, et al. Long-term outcomes for patients with solitary hepatocellular carcinoma treated by laparoscopic microwave coagulation. Cancer 2005;103(5):985–93.

53. Lencioni R, Crocetti L, Cioni D, et al. Percutaneous radiofrequency ablation of hepatic colorectal metastases: technique, indications, results, and new promises. Invest Radiol 2004;39(11):689–97.

54. Sperti E, Faggiuolo R, Gerbino A, et al. Outcome of metastatic colorectal cancer: analysis of a consecutive series of 229 patients. The impact of a multidisciplinary approach. Dis Colon Rectum 2006;49(10):1596–601.

55. Aloia TA, Vauthey JN, Loyer EM, et al. Solitary colorectal liver metastasis: resection determines outcome. Arch Surg 2006;141(5):460–6 [discussion: 466–7].

56. Wagner JS, Adson MA, Van Heerden JA, et al. The natural history of hepatic metastases from colorectal cancer. A comparison with resective treatment. Ann Surg 1984;199(5):502–8.

57. Scheele J, Stangl R, Altendorf-Hofmann A. Hepatic metastases from colorectal carcinoma: impact of surgical resection on the natural history. Br J Surg 1990; 77(11):1241–6.

58. Giovannini M. Percutaneous alcohol ablation for liver metastasis. Semin Oncol 2002;29(2):192–5.

59. Iannitti DA, Heniford T, Hale J, et al. Laparoscopic cryoablation of hepatic metastases. Arch Surg 1998;133(9):1011–5.

60. Siperstein AE, Berber E, Ballem N, et al. Survival after radiofrequency ablation of colorectal liver metastases: 10-year experience. Ann Surg 2007;246(4):559–65 [discussion: 565–7].

61. Sorensen SM, Mortensen FV, Nielsen DT. Radiofrequency ablation of colorectal liver metastases: long-term survival. Acta Radiol 2007;48(3):253–8.

62. Jakobs TF, Hoffmann RT, Trumm C, et al. Radiofrequency ablation of colorectal liver metastases: mid-term results in 68 patients. Anticancer Res 2006;26(1B): 671–80.

63. Liang P, Dong BW, Yu XL, et al. Evaluation of long-term therapeutic effects of ultrasound-guided percutaneous microwave ablation of liver metastases. Zhonghua Yi Xue Za Zhi 2006;86(12):806–10 [in Chinese].

64. Shibata T, Niinobu T, Ogata N, et al. Microwave coagulation therapy for multiple hepatic metastases from colorectal carcinoma. Cancer 2000;89(2):276–84.

65. Fong Y, Fortner J, Sun RL, et al. Clinical score for predicting recurrence after hepatic resection for metastatic colorectal cancer: analysis of 1001 consecutive cases. Ann Surg 1999;230(3):309–18 [discussion: 318–21].

66. Elias D, Benizri E, Pocard M, et al. Treatment of synchronous peritoneal carcinomatosis and liver metastases from colorectal cancer. Eur J Surg Oncol 2006; 32(6):632–6.

67. Weitz J, Blumgart LH, Fong Y, et al. Partial hepatectomy for metastases from non-colorectal, nonneuroendocrine carcinoma. Ann Surg 2005;241(2):269–76.

68. Knigge U, Hansen CP, Stadil F. Interventional treatment of neuroendocrine liver metastases. Surgeon 2008;6(4):232–9.

69. Greene FL. Carolinas Medical Center Surgical Teaching Program. Am Surg 2009; 75(12):1161–5.

Molecular Analysis of Breast Sentinel Lymph Nodes

Peter W. Blumencranz, MD[a],*, Maura Pieretti, PhD[b],
Kathleen G. Allen, MD[a], Lisa E. Blumencranz, BA[a]

KEYWORDS

- Breast cancer sentinel lymph node
- Molecular markers • PCR

DEVELOPMENT AND USE OF SENTINEL LYMPH NODE STAGING IN BREAST CANCER

The presence of metastatic disease in the axillary lymph nodes (ALNs) of patients with breast cancer has long been considered the most important prognostic factor for patients with newly diagnosed breast cancer.[1,2] The standard use of ALN dissection (ALND) has been to provide staging and prognostic information, as well as local control.

With vastly improved imaging techniques, primary breast cancer is being diagnosed earlier, at a smaller size, and with lower risk of having disease in the axilla. At present, approximately 24% of patients have positive nodes; therefore, the remainder derive no benefit from ALND.[3]

The development of lymphatic mapping and selective sentinel lymph node (SLN) lymphadenectomy has allowed many patients to be spared the sequelae of a full ALND, which would provide no therapeutic benefit but risk numerous side effects, including lymphedema, dysesthesias, and discomfort.[4]

Two major prospective studies as to the feasibility and accuracy of breast SLN biopsy were performed in National Surgical Adjuvant Breast and Bowel Project (NSABP) B-32 and the American College of Surgeons Oncology Group (ACOSOG) Z0010 trials. These trials encouraged the participation of community cancer centers such as the Morton Plant Hospital, thus providing the opportunity for community surgeons around the country to partner with their academic colleagues in major national trials. In Z0010, 29% of patients were enrolled from community practices.[5] SLN biopsy can identify for the pathologist those nodes most likely to contain

This work was supported in part by a grant from Veridex, LLC to Morton Plant Hospital.
[a] Comprehensive Breast Care Center of Tampa Bay, Morton Plant Hospital, 303 Pinellas Street, Clearwater, FL 33756, USA
[b] Molecular Diagnostic Laboratory, BayCare Laboratory, BayCare Health System, 210 Jeffords Street, Clearwater, FL 33756, USA
* Corresponding author.
E-mail address: peter.blumencranz@baycare.org

Surg Oncol Clin N Am 20 (2011) 467–485
doi:10.1016/j.soc.2011.01.002
1055-3207/11/$ – see front matter © 2011 Elsevier Inc. All rights reserved.

metastases. These few nodes can undergo a more thorough and labor-intensive analysis; however, there is no standardized protocol. It is commonly accepted that more sampling leads to an upstaging of the nodes (**Table 1**),[6–12] but evaluation is also subjective with interpretive disparity even among expert pathologists.[13,14]

Controversy also exists as to what size metastasis in a breast sentinel node is significant. The *American Joint Committee on Cancer* manual for cancer staging divides lymph node positivity into macrometastases 2 mm or greater, micrometastases 0.2 to less than 2 mm, and isolated tumor cells (ITCs). There is a relationship between the volume of disease in an SLN and the incidence of further axillary metastases (**Table 2**).[15–18] The general standard of care has been to complete an ALND for most patients with a positive SLN.[19] If the SLN status can be determined intraoperatively, the surgeon can complete the ALND at the time of the first surgery.

Current histologic methods for SLN evaluation have limitations. Histologic analysis on permanent section (PS) with hematoxylin and eosin (H&E) stain requires fixed tissue. This method is time consuming but allows high-quality morphologic analysis. PS has high specificity (99%–100%) and high sensitivity (85%–90%), but the latter depends on sampling thoroughness. Morphology is available, and size of metastases can be estimated. Unfortunately, there is no standard method for SLN processing and PS analysis. It is generally impractical to extensively sample each node for high sensitivity: usual methods examine only 2% to 5% of each node. PS is not intraoperative, and turnaround times vary greatly among different institutions. Histologic analysis requires an experienced pathologist, yet it still remains subjective. There are limitations identifying certain cancers such as lobular cell type. Immunohistochemistry (IHC) can be used in some cases to supplement PS analysis, especially to better identify cells expressing epithelial markers such as cytokeratins. However, IHC is not universally adopted, and there is no consensus as to its clinical significance.[19]

Intraoperative methods for SLN evaluation include frozen section (FS) and touch imprint cytology (TIC). FS has moderate sensitivity (57%–74%) with high specificity (99%–100%) (**Table 3**).[20–24] There is some morphologic information available and a rough estimate of the size of metastases. FS is usually available in 10 to 30 minutes intraoperatively. Again, there is no standard method for FS. It lacks higher sensitivity

Table 1		
Literature indicates more sampling finds more metastases		
Author, Year	**Increased H&E Cutting**	**Increase of Metastases Found (%)**
Treseler & Tauchi,[6] 2000	Multistudy summary	9–33
Yared et al,[7] 2002	One 5-μm level vs ten 5-μm levels	10
Liu et al,[8] 2000	1 level vs 3 additional H&E plus IHC	19
Cserni,[9] 2002	Five 5-μm levels (at 50–100 μm apart) vs complete node sectioning at 250 μm	19–28
Pargaonkar et al,[10] 2003	One 5-μm level vs 2 H&E and 3 IHC 5-μm levels	8
Motomura et al,[11] 2002	One 5 μm per node vs 1 level of H&E per 2 mm of node/additional H&E level plus IHC	3/16
Groen et al,[12] 2007	1 level per node half vs 3 levels, 150 μm apart per node half	12.5

Abbreviations: H&E, hematoxylin and eosin; IHC, immunohistochemistry.

Table 2
Incidence of further axillary metastasis predicted by size of SLN metastases

Size of SLN Metastasis	Incidence of Further Axillary Metastases (%)
>2 mm macrometastases	45–79
0.2 and <2 mm micrometastases	10–25
<0.2 mm submicrometastases	7–15
Negative	~10

Data from Refs.[15–18]

because sampling is limited, staining is less distinct, interpretation is even more subjective than PS, and certain cancers are difficult to identify, for example, lobular cancer. Other drawbacks of FS are loss of tissue in the microtome and freezing artifact on later PS analysis.

Like FS, TIC also has moderate sensitivity (45%–63%) with high specificity (98%–100%) (see **Table 3**).[24–27] There is no loss of tissue, and a 10- to 30-minute turnaround time allows intraoperative use. There is no standard method for TIC, and extensive sampling is not practical. TIC requires an expert cytopathologist, is subjective, is limited with the lobular subtype, and provides no size estimate. In a meta-analysis of sentinel node TIC in breast cancer by Tew and colleagues,[28] 31 studies were included, with a pooled sensitivity of 63% (95% confidence interval [CI], 57%–69%) and a specificity of 99% (95% CI, 98%–99%). Patients with invasive lobular cancer or micrometastases are more likely to have a false-negative finding.

The less-than-optimal sensitivity and the wide performance variability of current intraoperative methods for SLN evaluation often result in a delayed diagnosis and the need for a second surgery to perform ALND. The need for a more accurate intraoperative test, as well as a more objective, more reproducible, and less time-consuming postoperative test has spurred several investigations in the field of molecular analysis of SLNs.

DEVELOPMENT OF MOLECULAR MARKERS FOR SLN STAGING—A HISTORICAL PERSPECTIVE

Molecular analysis of breast SLNs emerged in the scientific and clinical literature in the late 1990s with many research studies initially focused on identifying suitable molecular markers for metastatic disease. Molecular analysis of the SLN consists of

Table 3
Current intraoperative tests are rapid, but lack sensitivity

Author, Year	Number of Cases	Method	Sensitivity (%)	Specificity (%)
Veronesi et al,[20] 1997	107	Frozen section	64	100
Rahusen et al,[21] 2000	106		57	100
Chao et al,[22] 2002	203		68	99
Tanis et al,[23] 2001	262		74	99
Creager,[24] 2002	646	Touch preparation	53	98
Dabbs,[25] 2004	748		45	99
Guldroz,[26] 2010	387		63	99
Komenaka,[27] 2010	107	Frozen section	74	100
		Touch preparation	61	100

studying gene expression at the messenger RNA (mRNA) level. Although the DNA of all genes is present in all cell types, only a few genes are expressed in any specific cell type with discrete production of mRNA and proteins. Theoretically, the detection of mRNA from genes not normally expressed in the lymph nodes indicates the presence of breast-derived cells or metastases.

Molecular analysis of the SLN involves extracting and purifying total mRNA from the homogenized lymph node followed by measuring mRNA levels of designated genes. Reverse transcription polymerase chain reaction (RT-PCR) produces a large number of copies of the chosen mRNA in vitro, which are then detected by gel electrophoresis (conventional RT-PCR) or by fluorescence measurement (real-time RT-PCR).

In general, molecular analysis has the potential to be more objective and reproducible than histologic analysis, as measuring gene expression is inherently less subjective than analyzing the morphology of cells. Because the entire node submitted is evaluated through the homogenization technique, molecular analysis evaluates more nodal tissue than typical histologic analysis, either intraoperatively or postoperatively.

In 1994, Schoenfeld and colleagues[29] found that the cytokeratin 19 (CK19) gene was a good discriminator differentiating those lymph nodes involved by breast cancer metastasis. Their analysis, which involved the lengthy process of RT-PCR followed by gel electrophoresis and hybridization, revealed superior sensitivity compared with the IHC analysis of CK19. Noguchi and colleagues[30] found that RT-PCR of the MUC1 and CK19 genes in an experimental setting allowed identification of 1 in 10^5 and 1 in 10^6 cancer cells, respectively. Using RT-PCR for MUC1 and CK19 to study pooled ALNs from 56 patients, gene expression was detected in 7 of the histologically negative patients and not detected in 1 histologically positive patient.

Both these initial studies as well as others[31–35] showed that molecular analysis could achieve higher sensitivity than histologic analysis. In light of this higher sensitivity, the realization that some level of expression of the genes chosen for molecular analysis could be present in normal lymph node cells raised concern about potential false-positive results.[36,37]

The melanoma-associated antigen 3 (MAGE-A3) marker sought to solve the specificity issue because this breast cancer gene is not expressed in any normal tissue. However, in the analysis by Wascher and colleagues,[38] only 45% of the histologically positive lymph nodes demonstrated MAGE-A3 expression. Therefore, although the specificity of this marker is potentially high, its low sensitivity precluded its further development into a clinical marker. Unfortunately, no specific marker for metastatic breast cancer has been reported to date.

In 2001, Manzotti and colleagues[39] evaluated 5 different genes in 146 SLNs from 123 patients and compared their expression with an extensive histologic analysis, which included 15 pairs of FS cut at 50- or 100-μm intervals for the entire length of the lymph node. Molecular analysis was performed on the intervening tissue slabs not used for histologic analysis. The sensitivity and specificity of the various markers varied, with MUC1 showing the highest specificity (100%) but the lowest sensitivity and mammoglobin (MG) showing the best combination of sensitivity (77.8%) and specificity (86%). The investigators concluded that the use of a multiple-marker RT-PCR assay had high concordance with an extensive histologic analysis. However, it was determined that further clinical follow-up of the patients was necessary to understand the full clinical implications of the molecular analysis.

All the molecular studies referenced up to this point used conventional RT-PCR. These studies often involved the use of nested PCR or a very large number of PCR cycles to improve sensitivity. These approaches have an inherent risk of contamination and only provide a qualitative analysis. The increasing use of real-time PCR in many laboratories in the early 2000s led to the development of more reproducible and quantitative assays. Real-time RT-PCR uses a closed tube system, reducing the risk of contamination. Real-time RT-PCR is quantitative and can discriminate between normal baseline gene expression and abnormally elevated gene expression such as found in the presence of metastases. Standardization of real-time PCR analyses can be accomplished by setting fixed analysis parameters and predetermined cutoffs.

In 2003, Inokuchi and colleagues[40] studied 358 ALNs from 22 patients using real-time RT-PCR. The expression of CK19 was compared with that of a normally expressed control gene. Cutoff values were first established by comparing the relative expression of CK19 in normal versus histologically positive lymph nodes. Using this method, 100% of the histologically positive and 9% of the histologically negative lymph nodes were positive by RT-PCR; furthermore, 3 of 4 histologically negative but IHC-positive nodes were positive by RT-PCR. This and other similar studies[41–44] started to highlight the potential for the use of real-time PCR in the molecular analysis of SLNs, as this method is less cumbersome than extensive sectioning of the node and can provide reproducible and quantifiable data.

Gillanders and colleagues[45] and Mikhitarian and colleagues[46] reported the findings of the MIMS (Minimally Invasive Molecular Staging of Breast Cancer) trial, a multi-institutional cohort study, where multimarker real-time RT-PCR analysis was applied to the analysis of SLNs and nonsentinel ALNs from 489 patients. The final report shows that the sensitivity of the combined pathologic and molecular SLN analysis to predict the metastatic status of ALNs was 92.8% compared with 84% for the pathologic analysis alone. The investigators also recognized the potential to tailor the molecular analysis so that the cutoff for positivity approximates the sensitivity of routine pathologic analysis or IHC.[46]

Another important aspect of real-time molecular assays is their suitability for intraoperative use because of the extreme speed of this type of PCR. Raja and colleagues[47] and Hughes and colleagues[48,49] reported the development of a completely automated cartridge-based molecular assay using the GeneXpert system in collaboration with the diagnostic company Cepheid (Sunnyvale, CA, USA). With this system, the cartridge is capable of performing nucleic acid isolation starting from a filtered lysate containing the SLN tissue. The cartridge, using lyophilized reagents and a microfluidics system, can automatically perform all the steps necessary for real-time RT-PCR and detection. The markers used in this system are 2 target genes (TACSTD1 and PIP) and an endogenous control gene. In their latest article,[49] the investigators report on the reproducibility studies performed at 3 different sites, as well as data for 29 positive and 30 negative control lymph nodes. Although the technical characteristics of this system are extremely intriguing, including the use of the bidirectional multiplexing strategy, it is unclear if any clinical studies have been initiated with this method.

In 2007, Tsujimoto and colleagues[50] reported the application of a novel assay, termed OSNA (one-step nucleic acid amplification), for the detection and quantitative measurement of CK19 mRNA in breast cancer lymph nodes. OSNA is based on a technology developed in 2000 called reverse transcription loop-mediated isothermal amplification.[51] With the OSNA assay, the lymph node tissue is solubilized and CK19 mRNA amplified without an intervening nucleic acid purification step. Amplification produces magnesium pyrophosphate, which is measured by turbidity. These features make OSNA a fast, simple technology that lends itself well to intraoperative use. The article by Tsujimoto and colleagues reports the establishment of cutoff values to distinguish macrometastases, micrometastases, and nonmetastases.[50] The analysis for cutoff calculations was based on PS and IHC performed on serial frozen sections taken at 10-μm intervals and OSNA performed on alternating node sections. Macrometastases had CK19 expression greater than 5×10^3 copies/μL, micrometastases had from 2.5×10^2 to 5×10^3 copies/μL, and nonmetastases had fewer than 2.5×10^2 copies/μL. Clinical validation studies to address the performance of OSNA compared with 3-level histopathologic analysis reported an overall 98% concordance in the 2007 article[50] and 93% concordance in a 2009 article by Tamaki and colleagues.[52] Despite the use of only 1 molecular marker and no internal control gene, Tamaki and colleagues reported a specificity of 94.3% and a sensitivity of 87.7% in a multi-institutional trial involving 164 patients in Japan. Visser and colleagues[53] evaluated OSNA in a study performed in the Netherlands on 32 patients and reported a sensitivity and specificity of 95.3% and 94.7%, respectively. Similar results were reported by Schem and colleagues[54] in 2009 in a German study. A 2-year prospective clinical study of OSNA was conducted in the United States from 2007 to 2008, and the results have been presented by Feldman[55] at the American Society of Breast Surgeons meeting in 2010. Results from 11 clinical sites evaluating 496 patients and 1044 SLNs showed an overall agreement between OSNA and reference pathology of 93.4% and 95.8% before and after discordant analysis, respectively. Sensitivity and specificity were 82.7% and 97.7%, respectively, after discordant analysis. Advantages of OSNA are its extreme speed and relative simplicity; the major disadvantage is that metastases of tumors not expressing CK19 are undetectable with this assay. OSNA indirectly allows the distinction between micrometastases and macrometastases, as the result of the test is reported as calculated CK19 copy number. This distinction potentially allows the surgeon to make an intraoperative decision regarding the performance of an ALND based on the size of the metastasis. The OSNA assay has received in vitro diagnostic product approval in Europe (CE mark) and in Asia and is commercially available through Sysmex (Mundelein, IL, USA).

Before the clinical development of the OSNA assay, Backus and colleagues[56] reported their investigation to identify optimal gene expression markers for breast cancer metastasis in SLN. This study is the basis for the development of the first US Food and Drug Administration (FDA)-approved assay commercially available in the United States: the GeneSearch Breast Lymph Node (BLN) Assay (Veridex, LLC, Warren, NJ, USA). The initial investigation involved a genome-wide gene expression analysis, as well as the study of 7 putative breast-specific markers and 1 internal control gene. After testing various marker combinations on histologically positive and negative lymph nodes, the investigators concluded that the gene pair with the highest sensitivity, at a specificity of 94%, was CK19 and MG. Porphobilinogen deaminase (PBGD) was chosen as the internal control gene because of its constant level of expression in lymph nodes.

A large multi-institutional clinical trial sponsored by Veridex followed this initial study and was performed between July 2004 and December 2005. The trial consisted of 2 separate clinical studies: the first included 304 patients at 12 US sites and determined the appropriate cutoff levels for CK19 and MG; the second included 416 patients at 11 US sites for the clinical validation of the assay. The Morton Plant Hospital participated in both studies, with the largest number of patients recruited and investigated at this site. These data have been published in detail previously[57–59] and are briefly reviewed here.

One of the major challenges of any molecular study of SLN is the appropriate calibration of the assay so that it does not detect clinically insignificant disease. For the BLN assay, the RT-PCR cutoffs were chosen so that micrometastases less than 0.2 mm would not yield positive results. Another challenge in the critical analysis of any molecular assay, including BLN, is that the tissue dedicated to molecular analysis is homogenized and therefore cannot be further analyzed morphologically. Any comparison between molecular and histologic analysis is therefore indirect, as it is performed on adjacent but not identical tissue portions. For the studies that led to the FDA approval of the BLN assay, PS analysis was considered the gold standard. To try to minimize sampling error, each node was sliced along the short axis into an even number of slabs 1.5 to 3 mm thick. The slabs used for histopathologic analysis were processed with PS, FS, or TIC as was standard at each institution and were used for patient management at each site. In addition, 3 extra PS slides were made from each tissue slab and were evaluated at a central pathology site; these slides consisted of three 4- to 6-μm thick sections collected at 3 levels, 150 μm apart.

In the validation series of 416 patients, when compared with PS, the assay detected 98% of metastases greater than 2 mm and 88% of metastases greater than 0.2 mm. Micrometastases were less frequently detected (57%), and assay-positive results in nodes found negative by histology were rare (4%). Disagreements seen between PS histology performed on adjacent node slabs and the molecular assay results were similar to the disagreements seen between histology performed on site slides versus central slides. Positive results of tests using additional molecular markers on nodes with positive BLN but overall negative histologic findings suggest that discrepancies were more likely due to sampling differences rather than to a false-positive result on BLN assay. In summary, the studies showed that BLN appeared to be a properly calibrated intraoperative molecular test that approaches the results obtained from PS histology. Compared with FS intraoperative testing, the assay showed improved sensitivity ranging from 10% to approximately 30%. In cases of invasive lobular carcinoma, FS sensitivity was 65.2% with a specificity of 97.8%, but the assay was 91.3% sensitive with a specificity of 95.7% (71 cases).

On July 17, 2007, the BLN assay received approval for clinical use from the FDA. The assay was labeled as a qualitative in vitro diagnostic test for the rapid detection of greater than 0.2 mm metastasis in nodal tissue removed from the sentinel node biopsies of breast cancer patients. Results from the assay could be used to guide intraoperative or postoperative decision making regarding removal of additional lymph nodes. The clinical use of the molecular assay began at Morton Plant Hospital on July 31, 2007. Analysis of that clinical use follows.

CLINICAL USE OF MOLECULAR MARKERS IN SLN STAGING

From July 31, 2007, until December 23, 2009, 478 consecutive patients with clinically node negative invasive breast cancer underwent lymphatic mapping and sentinel node biopsy at our institution. Patients consented to ALND to be performed at the time of the SLN biopsy if a node was found to be positive intraoperatively either by FS or by BLN. The FDA-approved cutting scheme and node sectioning method were used. Patients found to have node positivity only by postoperative PS had a second surgery for ALND. A retrospective review of these clinical data was conducted with written approval from our institutional review board. A total of 1111 SLNs were examined from 478 patients (average of 2.32 SLNs per patient).

Patient demographics are shown in **Table 4**. The average age was 62.5 years, and most had T1 tumors. About 74% underwent breast-conserving surgery. The overall histologic node positive rate was 17% (79 of 478), which is lower than in the clinical trials (28%). The possible explanations for the lower positive rate are the overall smaller tumor size and the increased use of preoperative axillary ultrasonography and lymph node needle biopsy, thereby precluding the need for SLN biopsy in some patients.

Table 4
Patient demographics and baseline characteristics

Age (y)	
Mean	62.55
Median	62
Range	29–92

Neoadjuvant therapy	
None	436
Received	42

Breast surgery	
Lumpectomy	355
Mastectomy	123

Primary invasive cancer	
Ductal	391
Lobular	46
Other	41

Tumor sizes (cm)	
Mean	1.57
Median	1.4
Range	0.0–6.0

Tumor grade (histologic)	
1	127
1–2	37
2	146
2–3	20
3	104
Unclassified	44

Estrogen receptor status	
Negative	151
Positive	327
Borderline	0

Progesterone receptor status	
Negative	229
Positive	246
Borderline	3

Human epidermal growth factor	
2 (HER2) status	
Negative	380
Positive	73
Borderline	25

Lymphovascular invasion	
Negative	347
Positive	27
Suspicious	17
Not reported	87

AJCC stage	
O[a]	17
I	307
IIA	109
IIB	26
IIIA	10
IIIB	2
IIIC	7

Abbreviation: AJCC, American Joint Committee on Cancer.
   [a] Received neoadjuvant treatment.
   Data from Morton Plant Hospital clinical use of the BLN assay.

Compared with PS, the BLN assay showed improved sensitivity over FS intraoperatively, with little loss in specificity (**Table 5**). The BLN assay was particularly helpful for tumors difficult to identify on FS as seen in the lobular type; the sensitivity was 100% (**Fig. 1**) and specificity was 94% (**Fig. 2**).

When an SLN was positive on the BLN assay, the ALND was positive in 40% of the cases. Only 4 patients had positive PS with a negative BLN, and none of these had a positive ALND. However, 33% of the patients with a negative FS had a positive ALND (**Table 6**).

Results were also analyzed by the size of metastases. If BLN was positive and PS negative, the ALND was still positive in 8 of 29 cases (28%), a rate similar to that for SLNs with micrometastases. On the contrary, if FS was positive and PS was negative (3 cases), the ALND was always negative (**Table 7**).

A timing study was also conducted to see how long it took to receive the BLN assay results from the laboratory, measuring the interval from the time the nodes were sent from the operating room until the results were called to the surgeon. Results were available generally in 30 to 35 minutes, with few surgical delays more than 5 minutes (**Fig. 3**).

Further analysis of this series was presented at the 11th Annual Meeting of the American Society of Breast Surgeons in May 2010 to see the effect on reduction in second surgeries.[60] From January 2005 to July 2007 (pre-BLN), 52 of 156 patients (33%) required to be taken back to the operating room for completion ALND because of false-negative results from FS. From July 2007 to December 2009 (both FS and BLN used), only 8 of 151 patients (5%) required such second surgery. The percentage of patients in both periods needing ALND was essentially the same: 21% (156 of 736) pre-BLN and 20% (151 of 767) post-BLN. This result suggests that the BLN assay was not too sensitive, causing unnecessary ALNDs; it is better that patients received their operation at the initial surgery with less stress on the patient, family, and medical staff, as well as lower overall cost.

Our data are similar to those of several publications reporting the clinical use of the BLN assay in different countries.[61–65] Findings of the major studies are summarized in **Table 8**. All investigators used the BLN assay for clinical decision making, although not all intraoperatively. Most followed the recommended SLN cutting scheme and compared the BLN results with PS results. An exception was the study by Tafe and colleagues,[65] in which only tissue from the outer parts of the SLN was submitted for BLN assay. Viale and colleagues,[61] on the other hand, followed the recommended BLN cutting scheme but performed a more extensive analysis of the SLN by PS. As expected, in the latter report, the sensitivity of BLN was lower compared with the other reports, as more metastases were found by analyzing the SLN by PS in its entirety. Most investigators who have used the BLN assay in a clinical setting concur that it can detect macrometastases with extreme sensitivity, such as 100% in the studies by Mansel and colleagues[63] and Cutress and colleagues[64] and 98% in the study by Viale and

Table 5					
Performance compared with PS					
Test Method	**Number of Patients**	**Sensitivity (%)**	**Specificity (%)**	**PPV (%)**	**NPV (%)**
Frozen Section	4.78	66	99	95	94
BLN Assay		95	93	72	99

Abbreviations: NPV, negative predictive value; PPV, positive predictive value.
Data from Morton Plant Hospital clinical use of BLN assay.

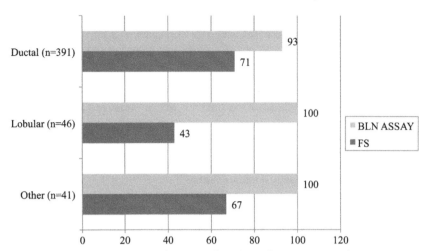

Fig. 1. BLN assay and FS sensitivity by cancer histological type compared to PS.

colleagues.[61] As expected, micrometastases were detected across the different sites with lower sensitivity because of larger sampling variability with smaller tumor deposits.

The reproducibility of data generated with the BLN assay across different sites is also evident from the combined analysis of 1138 patients from 4 US sites, including our institution, 1 Belgium site, and 1 UK site as presented at the Improving Care and Knowledge through Translational Research Breast Cancer Conference on May 7, 2009, in Brussels.[66] Assay turnaround times were similar as were positive rates, sensitivity, and specificity. The analysis of this large series of patients also showed an excellent negative predictive value (NPV) for the presence of disease in the ALND. NPV of the BLN assay alone was 96% and of BLN and PS combined was 99%. This high NPV assures the patient, the surgeon, and the pathologist that occult metastases are unlikely.

The BLN assay has been approved for clinical use as a qualitative assay; however, it is a real-time PCR assay capable of quantitative results. Although not visible to the

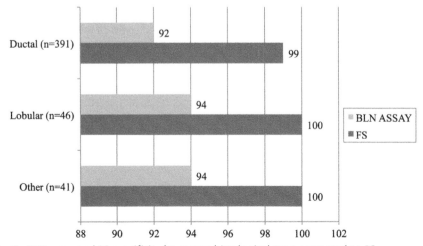

Fig. 2. BLN assay and FS specificity by cancer histological type compared to PS.

Table 6
BLN/FS SLN prediction of node positivity in ALND

SLN Status			ALN Status	
Intraoperative Result	Histology SLN (H&E)	Number of Patients	# Performed	# Positive (%)
BLN assay				
Negative	Negative	370	ND	N/A
	Positive	4	4	0 (0%)
Positive	Negative	29	29	8 (28%)
	Positive	75	75	34 (45%)
Frozen section				
Negative	Negative	396	28	8 (29%)
	Positive	27	27	11 (41%)
Positive	Negative	3	3	0 (0%)
	Positive	52	52	23 (44%)

Data from Morton Plant Hospital clinical use of BLN assay.

operator using the FDA-approved software, quantitative data are generated for each of the markers measured (CK19, MG, and PBGD). Gene expression is measured by the fluorescent detection of the amplification product during RT-PCR and reported as a Ct (cycle threshold) value: the higher the level of a target gene mRNA the lower the Ct (**Fig. 4**). Confirming the quantitative nature of the BLN assay, both Veys and colleagues[67] and Viale and colleagues[61] reported a reverse association between metastasis size and Ct values for CK19 and MG. We presented similar data on our series at the San Antonio Breast Conference in 2008[68] and showed a high level of correlation ($r = 0.74$ for MG and 0.72 for CK19, $P<.0001$). In addition, we showed that lower Ct values were also correlated to the probability of non-SLN positivity, with 74% of cases with CK19 Ct less than or equal to 24 and MG Ct less than or equal to 32 having at least 1 positive lymph node from ALND.

Our institution also conducted 2 analyses to integrate the information from the BLN assay with other factors commonly used in nomograms such as age, tumor size, grade, and ER/PR/HER2 status.[69,70] In the study by Chagpar and colleagues,[70] 728 patients from 2 clinical sites were analyzed. A BLN score including the Ct values of

Table 7
BLN/FS SLN prediction by size of metastasis

SLN Status		ALN Status	
Histology SLN (H&E)	Number of Patients	# Performed	# Positive (%)
BLN assay positives			
Macrometastases (>2 mm)	42	42	22 (52%)
Micrometastases (0.2–2 mm)	33	33	12 (36%)
Negative	29	29	8 (28%)
Frozen section positives			
Macrometastases (>2 mm)	38	38	18 (47%)
Micrometastases (0.2–2 mm)	14	14	5 (36%)
Negative	3	3	0 (0%)

Data from Morton Plant Hospital clinical use of BLN assay.

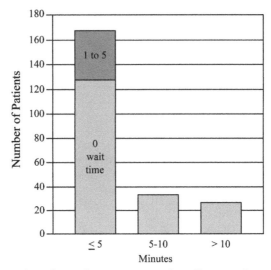

Fig. 3. BLN assay timing data. The average runtime (from node removal to surgeon receiving the results) is 37 minutes. Figure shows the length of time, in minutes, the surgeon had to wait for the BLN assay result from when the breast surgery was completed. About 72% of the time the surgeon did not need to wait more than 5 minutes for the assay result.

MG and CK19 and the number of nodes positive by BLN assay was a significant predictor of non-SLN metastases. When the BLN score was combined with other information that is available intraoperatively such as tumor size and proportion of SLN positivity by FS or TIC, the estimation of non-SLN metastases was quite accurate (62.5% of non-SLNs were positive with a high score, whereas <5% were positive with a low score). These data show that the quantitative information from the BLN assay results, in combination with other clinical information, could be used to better tailor the surgeon's decision to perform ALND at the time of the first surgery.

As of late December 2009, Veridex decided to remove the BLN assay from the worldwide commercial market. This was not because of poor clinical performance of the assay but because of lack of early adoption. At present, there is no commercially available FDA-approved molecular assay for SLN. However, the OSNA assay distributed by Sysmex is available abroad.

Table 8
Clinical use of the BLN assay

Author	Clinical Sites	Number of Patients	Positive by BLN Assay (%)	Sensitivity vs PS (%)	Specificity vs PS (%)
Viale et al,[61] 2008	Milan, Italy	293	22.8	77.8	95.0
Veys et al,[62] 2009	Brussels, Belgium	367	19.6	89.0	94.5
Mansel et al,[63] 2009	Cardiff, UK	82	14.6	88.9	94.6
Cutress et al,[64] 2010	Portsmouth, UK	254	30.7	96.0	95.0
Tafe et al,[65] 2010	Dartmouth, NH, USA	59	18.6	88.9	93.5
Blumencranz et al [this article]	Clearwater, FL, USA	478	21.7	95.0	93.0

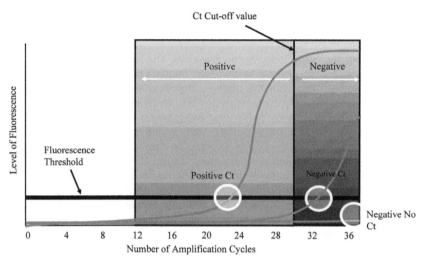

Fig. 4. GeneSearch BLN assay: qualitative interpretation. Typical real-time PCR growth curves are show with gray lines; when the line crosses the fluorescence threshold, a Ct value is determined based on cycle number. If Ct is lower than the established cutoff, the PCR reaction is positive. Ct cutoff values in the BLN assay are 30 for CK19 and 31 for MG. (*Courtesy of* Veridex, LLC, Raritan, NJ, USA; with permission.)

CONTROVERSIES AND SUMMARY

Although there is accumulating data regarding the reproducibility and reliability of molecular assessment of sentinel nodes, there are still several controversies. At present, there are no specific markers for breast cancer cells, and the markers that are currently used reflect the presence of breast tissue or epithelial tissue, such as CK19 expression. Because these markers are not specific for metastatic breast cells, there is concern in the literature about false-positive results caused by displaced cells. There is concern that iatrogenic epithelial cell displacement and benign transport of breast epithelial cells into axillary nodes could cause a false-positive molecular result that cannot be verified morphologically because the portion analyzed by the molecular assay has been homogenized.[71] In the study by Bleiweiss and colleagues,[71] 25 cases were reported, with 22 patients having coincidental papillomas and 15 with ductal carcinoma in situ (DCIS) only. These 25 cases had cytokeratin-positive SLNs but contained single cells or clusters with 1 to 35 cells. The number of cells required for the BLN molecular assay to be positive far exceeds this number, and as calibrated, it is estimated to be in the range of 2000 cells.[58] It is also of interest that in the BLN clinical trial with a total of 722 patients, none had benign epithelial cells reported in the sentinel nodes. The study by Bleiweiss and colleagues[71] concludes that one should not do a sentinel node dissection, particularly for cases of DCIS involving intraductal papilloma. In fact, the FDA approval for the BLN assay was for invasive breast cancer only. If one considers doing lymphatic mapping and sentinel node biopsy in a case of high-grade or more-extensive DCIS, it is inadvisable to perform either IHC staining or molecular study on those sentinel nodes.

Another controversial point is the loss of morphology. The portion of the node homogenized for molecular assay cannot yield morphology. Extranodal extension cannot be derived in tissue submitted for molecular analysis. It can be argued that a positive molecular test result represents numerous ITCs with no cluster greater than 0.2 mm. However, if the number of ITCs is sufficient to generate a positive PCR result, one could argue that the molecular analysis is more accurate in determining the true tumor burden in the node.

Some consider molecular assays too sensitive, but in our overall series of 478 cases, there were numerous instances in which sentinel nodes in the slabs preserved for histology showed ITCs, but the slabs composing the other 50% of the node showed negative results on molecular evaluation, even in patients in whom another node was positive on histology and molecular analysis. This finding suggests that the Ct values were calibrated appropriately. Viale and colleagues[61] from Milan did a comparative evaluation of the BLN assay and an extensive histopathologic examination of the SLNs by studying a prospective series of 293 consecutive SLNs from 293 patients. Extensive histopathologic evaluation was performed on serial frozen sections cut at 40- to 50-μm intervals. All the 50-μm interval tissue were retrieved and subjected to RT-PCR assay, with the alternate pieces discarded to mimic the way the nodes would be handled according to the BLN protocol. This analysis allowed a more accurate estimate of the true histologic size of the metastasis in each node relative to the results of the BLN assay. The metastatic deposit for BLN positivity was estimated to be 0.8 mm, significantly more than the 0.2 mm cutoff for micrometastatic disease. The BLN assay has comparable sensitivity to extensive histopathologic examination, with much less time, effort, and cost.

In our clinical use (N = 478), we found very few patients whose sentinel nodes were positive on molecular analysis, but negative on histologic analysis. In 8 of 29 (28%) such patients, positive nodes were detected in the axilla after ALND, suggesting that the molecular assay identified true disease. It is impossible to state with certainty that all nodes that are positive on molecular analysis and negative on histologic analysis do not contain some type of displaced cell or epithelial inclusion. However, it is unlikely that displaced cells would be at such levels to create a positive result in the BLN assay.

Further widespread controversy exists about the entire issue of the significance of micrometastases or ITCs. Micrometastases are certainly associated with the risk of additional nonsentinel node positivity as cited earlier in this article. What is not clear is the associated risk for systemic recurrence and local regional recurrence or the benefit of completing ALND. The clinical standard has traditionally been completion of ALND, but already many surgeons are not completing ALND, especially for micrometastatic disease.[72] At the 2010 Annual Meeting of the American Surgical Association, Giuliano and colleagues[73] presented a 5-year follow-up study from the ACOSOG Z0011 prospective randomized trial examining survival of patients with sentinel node metastasis detected by standard H&E and treated with and without ALND or axillary radiation. Local and regional recurrence was evaluated. A total of 446 patients received sentinel node biopsy alone, with no more than 2 sentinel nodes positive and no extranodal extension or matted nodes, and 445 patients were randomized to a sentinel node biopsy followed by completion ALND. There was a median follow-up of 5.9 years. Differences in neither the local recurrence nor regional recurrence were statistically significant between the 2 groups. The conclusion, despite the potential of residual disease in the axilla, is that sentinel node biopsy alone can offer excellent regional control and may be a reasonable management for selected patients with breast cancer. The Z0011 trial, however, excluded many patients, for example, those undergoing mastectomy without radiotherapy, partial-breast irradiation, preoperative neoadjuvant therapy, or whole-breast irradiation in the prone position, who, at this point, should not be denied ALND.

In view of the changing clinical significance of metastatic disease in SLNs and the diminished role for ALND, the need for improved intraoperative evaluation of the

SLN is in question. The challenges related to the lack of sensitivity of current methods, as well as the lack of standardization of routine histologic analyses still remain. Molecular assays, however, offer one way to standardize such analyses. When calibrated to clinically significant cutoffs, they can provide excellent reproducibility, objective results, and lower cost. Molecular assays of the sentinel node could be used as an adjunct to histologic analyses, or the whole node could be homogenized to give a better estimate of the tumor burden in the SLNs. This concept would likely be more accepted if there were further studies on the correlation between quantitative RT-PCR and volume of tumor.

Recent data suggest that ALND may not be needed for early-stage primary tumors with low nodal involvement, but there is still a role for sentinel node biopsy in all patients with invasive breast cancer. At present, available molecular signatures on the primary tumor used for prognosis and prediction have been applied mainly in node negative patients. Although there may be a time when these gene profiles are so accurate in guiding treatment that node status for prognosis may be irrelevant, this is not as yet. Therefore, accurate staging of the SLN still has a role. Furthermore, there are many sites in the world where qualified breast pathologists are not available, and affordable molecular platforms for sentinel node analysis could allow accurate assessment of sentinel nodes by a trained technologist. Our clinical experience with one of these assays supports the accuracy of molecular staging and gives a preview of the potential use of this platform in other solid tumors with discovery of appropriate markers.

REFERENCES

1. Fisher B, Bauer M, Wickersham DC, et al. Relationship of number of positive axillary nodes to the prognosis of patients with primary breast cancer. Cancer 1983; 52:1551–7.
2. Fisher ER, Sass E, Fisher B, et al. Pathologic findings from the NSABP protocol 4: discriminates for tenth year treatment failure. Cancer 1984;53:712–23.
3. Bilimoria KY, Bentrem DJ, Hansen NM, et al. Comparison of sentinel lymph node biopsy alone and completion axillary node dissection for node-positive breast cancer. J Clin Oncol 2009;27:2946–53.
4. Petrek JA, Senie RT, Peters M, et al. Lymphedema in a cohort of breast carcinoma survivors 20 years after diagnosis. Cancer 2001;92:1368–77.
5. Leitch AM, Beitsch PD, McCall LM, et al. Patterns of participation and successful patient recruitment to American College of Surgeons Oncology Group Z0010, a phase II trial for patients with early-stage breast cancer. Am J Surg 2005;190:539–42.
6. Treseler PA, Tauchi PS. Pathologic analysis of the sentinel node. Surg Clin North Am 2000;80:1695–719.
7. Yared MA, Middleton LP, Smith TL, et al. Recommendations for sentinel lymph node processing in breast cancer. Am J Surg Pathol 2002;26:377–82.
8. Liu LH, Siziopikou KP, Gabram S, et al. Evaluation of axillary sentinel lymph node biopsy by immunohistochemistry and multilevel sectioning in patients with breast carcinoma. Arch Pathol Lab Med 2000;124:1670–3.
9. Cserni G. Complete sectioning of axillary sentinel nodes in patients with breast cancer. Analysis of two different step sectioning and immunohistochemistry protocols in 246 patients. J Clin Pathol 2002;55:926–31.
10. Pargaonkar AS, Beissner RS, Snyder S, et al. Evaluation of immunohistochemistry and multiple-level sectioning in sentinel lymph nodes from patients with breast cancer. Arch Pathol Lab Med 2003;127:701–5.

11. Motomura K, Komoike Y, Inaji H, et al. Multiple sectioning and immunohistochemical staining of sentinel nodes in patients with breast cancer. Br J Surg 2002;89: 1032–4.

12. Groen RS, Oosterhuis AW, Boers JE. Pathologic examination of sentinel lymph nodes in breast cancer by a single haematoxylin-eosin slide versus serial sectioning and immunocytokeratin staining: clinical implications. Breast Cancer Res Treat 2007;105:1–5.

13. Roberts CA, Beitsch PD, Litz CE. Interpretative disparity among pathologists in breast sentinel lymph node evaluation. Am J Surg 2003;186:324–9.

14. Cserni G. What is a positive sentinel node in a breast cancer patient? A practical approach. Breast 2007;16:152–60.

15. Degnim AC, Griffith KA, Sabel MS, et al. Clinicopathologic features of metastasis in nonsentinel lymph nodes of breast carcinoma patients. Cancer 2003;98: 2307–15.

16. van Rijk MC, Peterse JL, Niewig OE, et al. Additional axillary metastases and stage migration in breast cancer patients with micrometastases or submicrometastases in sentinel lymph nodes. Cancer 2006;107:467–71.

17. Viale G, Maiorano E, Mazzarol G, et al. Histologic detection and clinical implications of micrometastases in axillary sentinel lymph nodes for patients with breast carcinoma. Cancer 2001;92:1378–84.

18. Cserni G, Amendoeira I, Apostolikas N, et al. Pathological work up of sentinel lymph nodes in breast cancer. Review of current data to be considered for the formulation of guidelines. Eur J Cancer 2003;39:1654–67.

19. Silverstein MJ, Recht A, Lagios M, et al. Special report: consensus conference III. Image-detected breast cancer: state-of-the-art diagnosis and treatment. J Am Coll Surg 2009;209:504–20.

20. Veronesi U, Paganelli G, Galimberti V, et al. Sentinel-node biopsy to avoid axillary dissection in breast cancer with clinically negative lymph-nodes. Lancet 1997; 349:1864–7.

21. Rahusen FD, Pijpers R, Van Diest PJ, et al. The implementation of the sentinel node biopsy as a routine procedure for patients with breast cancer. Surgery 2000;128:6–12.

22. Chao C, Wong SL, Ackermann D, et al. Utility of intraoperative frozen section analysis of sentinel lymph nodes in breast cancer. Am J Surg 2001;182:609–15.

23. Tanis PJ, Boom RP, Koops HS, et al. Frozen section investigation of the sentinel node in malignant melanoma and breast cancer. Ann Surg Oncol 2001;8:222–6.

24. Creager AJ, Geisinger KR, Shiver SA, et al. Intraoperative evaluation of sentinel lymph nodes for metastatic breast carcinoma by imprint cytology. Mod Pathol 2002;15:1140–7.

25. Dabbs DJ, Fung M, Johnson R. Intraoperative cytologic examination of breast sentinel lymph nodes: test utility and patient impact. Breast J 2004;10:190–4.

26. Guldroz JA, Johnson MT, Scott-Conner C, et al. The use of touch preparation for the evaluation of sentinel nodes in breast cancer. Am J Surg 2010;199:792–6.

27. Komenaka IK, Torabi R, Nair G, et al. Intraoperative touch imprint and frozen section analysis of sentinel lymph nodes after neoadjuvant chemotherapy for breast cancer. Ann Surg 2010;251:319–22.

28. Tew K, Irwig L, Mattews A, et al. Meta-analysis of sentinel node imprint cytology in breast cancer. Br J Surg 2005;92:1068–80.

29. Schoenfeld A, Luqmani Y, Smith D, et al. Detection of breast cancer micrometastases in axillary lymph nodes by using polymerase chain reaction. Cancer Res 1994;54:2986–90.

30. Noguchi S, Aihara T, Motomura K, et al. Detection of breast cancer micrometastases in axillary lymph nodes by means of reverse transcriptase-polymerase chain
reaction. Am J Pathol 1996;148:649–56.
31. Mori M, Mimori K, Inoue H, et al. Detection of cancer micrometastases in lymph
nodes by reverse transcriptase-polymerase chain reaction. Cancer Res 1995;55:
3417–20.
32. Bostick PJ, Huynh KT, Sarantou T, et al. Detection of metastases in sentinel lymph
nodes of breast cancer patients by multiple-marker RT-PCR. Int J Cancer 1998;
79:645–51.
33. Min CJ, Tafra L, Verbanac KM. Identification of superior markers for polymerase
chain reaction detection of breast cancer metastases in sentinel lymph nodes.
Cancer Res 1998;58:4581–4.
34. Aihara T, Fujiwara Y, Ooka M, et al. Mammaglobin B as a novel marker for detection
of breast cancer micrometastases in axillary lymph nodes by reverse transcription-
polymerase chain reaction. Breast Cancer Res Treat 1999;58:137–40.
35. Masuda N, Tamaki Y, Sakita I, et al. Clinical significance of micrometastases in
axillary lymph nodes assessed by reverse transcription-polymerase chain reaction in breast cancer patients. Clin Cancer Res 2000;6:4176–85.
36. Yun K, Gunn J, Merrie AE, et al. Keratin 19 mRNA is detectable by RT-PCR in
lymph nodes of patients without breast cancer. Br J Cancer 1997;76:1112–3.
37. Ruud P, Fodstad O, Hovig E. Identification of a novel cytokeratin 19 pseudogene
that may interfere with reverse transcriptase-polymerase chain reaction assays
used to detect micrometastatic tumor cells. Int J Cancer 1999;80:119–25.
38. Wascher RA, Bostick PJ, Huyn KT, et al. Detection of MAGE-A3 in breast cancer
patients' sentinel lymph nodes. Br J Cancer 2001;85:1340–8.
39. Manzotti M, Dell'Orto P, Maisonneuve P, et al. Reverse transcription-polymerase
chain reaction assay for multiple mRNA markers in the detection of breast cancer
metastases in sentinel lymph nodes. Int J Cancer 2001;95:307–12.
40. Inokuchi M, Ninomiya U, Tsugawa K, et al. Quantitative evaluation of metastases
in axillary lymph nodes of breast cancer. Br J Cancer 2003;89:1750–6.
41. Zehenter BK, Dillon DC, Jiang Y, et al. Application of a multigene RT-PCR assay
for the detection of mammoglobin and complementary transcribed genes in
breast cancer lymph nodes. Clin Chem 2002;48:1225–31.
42. Sakaguchi M, Virmani A, Dudak MW, et al. Clinical relevance of reverse transcrip-
tase polymerase chain reaction for the detection of axillary lymph node metastases in breast cancer. Ann Surg Oncol 2003;10:117–25.
43. Weigelt B, Verdujin P, Bosma AJ, et al. Detection of metastases in sentinel lymph
nodes of breast cancer patients by multiple mRNA markers. Br J Cancer 2004;90:
1531–7.
44. Nissan A, Jager D, Roystacher M, et al. Multimarker RT-PCR assay for the detection of minimal residual disease in sentinel lymph nodes of breast cancer
patients. Br J Cancer 2006;94:681–5.
45. Gillanders WE, Mikhitarian K, Hebert R, et al. Molecular detection of micrometastatic breast cancer in histopathology-negative axillary lymph nodes correlates
with traditional predictors of prognosis. An interim analysis of a prospective
multi-institutional cohort study. Ann Surg 2004;239:828–40.
46. Mikhitarian K, Hebert Martin R, Mitas M, et al. Molecular analysis improves sensitivity of breast sentinel lymph node biopsy: results of a multi-institutional prospective cohort study. Surgery 2005;138:474–80.
47. Raja S, Ching J, Xi L, et al. Technology for automated, rapid and quantitative PCR
or reverse transcription PCR clinical testing. Clin Chem 2005;51:882–90.

48. Hughes SJ, Liqiang X, Raja S, et al. A rapid, fully automated, molecular-based assay accurately analyzes sentinel lymph nodes for the presence of metastatic breast cancer. Ann Surg 2006;143:389–98.

49. Hughes SJ, Liqiang X, Gooding WE, et al. A quantitative reverse transcription PCR assay for rapid, automated analysis of breast cancer sentinel lymph nodes. J Mol Diagn 2009;11:576–82.

50. Tsujimoto M, Nakabayashi K, Yoshidome K, et al. One-step nucleic acid amplification for intraoperative detection of lymph node metastasis in breast cancer patients. Clin Cancer Res 2007;13:4807–16.

51. Notomi T, Okayama H, Masubuchi H, et al. Loop-mediated isothermal amplification of DNA. Nucleic Acids Res 2000;28:E63.

52. Tamaki Y, Akiyama F, Iwase T, et al. Molecular detection of lymph node metastases in breast cancer patients: results of a multicenter trial using the one-step nucleic acid amplification assay. Clin Cancer Res 2009;15:2879–84.

53. Visser M, Jiwa M, Horstman A, et al. Intra-operative diagnostic method based on CK19 mRNA expression for the detection of lymph node metastases in breast cancer. Int J Cancer 2008;122:2562–7.

54. Schem C, Maass N, Bauerschlag DO, et al. One-step nucleic acid amplification– a molecular method for the detection of lymph node metastases in breast cancer patients; results of the German study group. Virchows Arch 2009;454:203–10.

55. Feldman S, Krishnamurthy S, Gillanders W, et al. A novel automated assay for the rapid identification of metastatic breast carcinoma in sentinel lymph nodes. Cancer 2011. [Epub ahead of print].

56. Backus J, Laughlin T, Wang Y, et al. Identification and characterization of optimal gene expression markers for detection of breast cancer metastasis. J Mol Diagn 2005;7:327–36.

57. Blumencranz P, Deck KB, Whitworth PW, et al. Clinical evaluation of a molecular assay for the detection of metastases in breast sentinel lymph nodes. Arch Pathol Lab Med 2006;130:1362.

58. Blumencranz P, Whitworth P, Deck K, et al. Sentinel node staging for breast cancer: intra-operative molecular pathology overcomes conventional histologic sampling errors. Am J Surg 2007;194:426–32.

59. Julian T, Blumencranz P, Deck K, et al. Novel intraoperative molecular test for sentinel lymph node metastasis with patients with early-stage breast cancer. J Clin Oncol 2008;26:3338–45.

60. Blumencranz P, Pieretti M, Blumencranz L. Reduction in second surgeries for axillary lymph node dissection in breast cancer patients using an intraoperative RT-PCR assay. In: Official Proceedings of the 11th Annual Meeting of the American Society of Breast Surgeons. Las Vegas (NV): 2010. p. 10.

61. Viale G, Dell'Orto P, Biasi MO, et al. Comparative evaluation of an extensive histopathologic examination and a real-time reverse-transcription-polymerase chain reaction assay for mammoglobin and cytokeratin 19 on axillary sentinel nodes of breast carcinoma patients. Ann Surg 2008;247(1):1–7.

62. Veys I, Durbecq V, Majjaj S, et al. Eighteen months clinical experience with the GeneSearch breast lymph node assay. Am J Surg 2009;198:203–9.

63. Mansel RE, Goyal A, Douglas-Jones A, et al. Detection of breast cancer metastasis in sentinel lymph nodes using intra-operative real time GeneSearch™ BLN Assay in the operating room: results of the Cardiff study. Breast Cancer Res Treat 2009;115:595–600.

64. Cutress RI, McDowell A, Gabriel FG, et al. Observational and cost analysis of the implementation of breast cancer sentinel node intraoperative molecular diagnosis. J Clin Pathol 2010;63:522–9.
65. Tafe LJ, Schwab MC, Lefferts JA, et al. A validation study of a new molecular diagnostic assay: the Dartmouth-Hitchcock Medical Center experience with the GeneSearch BLN assay in breast sentinel nodes. Exp Mol Pathol 2010;88:1–6.
66. Larsimont D, Durbecq V, Veys I, et al. Prediction of axillary status from sentinel lymph node testing with an intra-operative RT-PCR test–multi-center analysis of 1138 patients. Ann Oncol 2009;20:22.
67. Veys I, Majjaj S, Salgado R, et al. Evaluation of the histological size of the sentinel lymph node metastases using RT-PCR assay: a rapid tool to estimate the risk of non-sentinel lymph node invasion in patients with breast cancer. Breast Cancer Res Treat 2009;124:599–605.
68. Blumencranz P, Pieretti M, Hasad H, et al. Quantitative intra-operative RT-PCR assay predicts size of sentinel node metastases. Cancer Res 2009;69(Suppl):1002.
69. Blumencranz P, Pieretti M. Rapid molecular RT-PCR assay to detect metastases in sentinel lymph nodes of breast cancer patients may accurately predict further axillary positivity. Cancer Res 2009;69(Suppl):1016.
70. Chagpar AB, Blumencranz P, Whitworth PW, et al. Use of pre- and intra-operative data to predict probability of positive non-sentinel lymph nodes. Cancer Res 2009;302(Suppl):302.
71. Bleiweiss IJ, Nagi CS, Jaffer S. Axillary sentinel lymph nodes can be falsely positive due to iatrogenic displacement and transport of benign epithelial cells in patients with breast carcinoma. J Clin Oncol 2008;24:2013–8.
72. Wasif N, Maggard MA, Ko CY, et al. Underuse of axillary dissection for the management of sentinel node micrometastases in breast cancer. Arch Surg 2010;145:161–6.
73. Giuliano AE, McCall L, Beitsch P, et al. Locoregional recurrence after sentinel lymph node dissection with or without axillary dissection in patients with sentinel lymph node metastases: the American College of Surgeons Oncology group Z 0011 randomized trial. Ann Surg 2010;252:426–32.

Pancreatic Resection in a Large Tertiary Care Community-Based Hospital: Building a Successful Pancreatic Surgery Program

Ryan Z. Swan, MD, Kwan N. Lau, MD, David Sindram, MD, PhD, David A. Iannitti, MD, John B. Martinie, MD*

KEYWORDS

- Pancreatic resection • Pancreatic cancer • Pancreatectomy
- Community hospital • Outcomes

Pancreatic cancer is the fourth leading cause of cancer death in the United States, with more than 43,000 new cases and 36,800 deaths estimated in 2010 alone.[1] The 5-year survival rate for patients with pancreatic cancer remains less than 5%.[1] Because curative systemic treatment modalities for pancreatic cancer have yet to be discovered, pancreatic resection remains the only potentially curative treatment option for the less-unfortunate one of five patients with a resectable lesion. For these patients, a combination of surgical resection with adjuvant chemotherapy can provide a 5-year survival rate of up to 30%.[2]

Delivery of the highest quality surgical care to patients with pancreatic cancer requires considerable dedication of hospital resources, specific expertise, and inter-departmental coordination.[3,4] Therefore, the appropriate setting for pancreatic surgery has been a topic of intense debate recently.[5,6] Most current evidence suggests that hospitals with a high annual volume of pancreatic surgeries have improved short- and long-term risk-adjusted outcomes after pancreatic resection

Conflict of interest: The authors have nothing to disclose.
Hepato-Pancreato-Biliary Surgery, Department of General Surgery, Carolinas Medical Center, 1025 Morehead Medical Plaza Drive, Suite 300, Charlotte, NC 28204, USA
* Corresponding author.
E-mail address: john.martinie@carolinashealthcare.org

for cancer.[7–16] Experts have proposed that higher volume is likely a definable surrogate marker for higher-quality systems of patient care at these centers.[5,6]

Given these data, regionalization of pancreatic resections to high-volume centers seems ideal; however, significant obstacles remain, including disparities in access to a high-volume center, prolonged patient travel times, patient preference for local over remote care, and the impact of a referral policy on the referring and receiving hospitals.[4,17–20] Despite these limitations, significant steps have been taken in the United States and Europe toward regionalization of pancreatic resection[7,11,12,20–22]; nevertheless, most pancreatic resections in the United States are still performed at low- or medium-volume centers.[4,11,17]

Most of these high-volume centers are large, academic, tertiary care hospitals, and the low- and medium-volume centers are essentially community hospitals of varying size with or without an academic affiliation. In response to the large volume of literature showing better outcomes at high-volume centers, surgeons at many of these low- to medium-volume community hospitals have published their exceptional outcomes after pancreatic resection.[23–27] A cohesive argument has been made that volume does not dictate outcome; however, high-volume centers on average operate significantly higher-quality systems of care, and these systems do dictate outcome.[3,5,6] Significant efforts have been made to understand the structure and process behind this association, with the hope that these systems can translate into improved patient care at low- and medium-volume centers.[3,28–30] Multiple preoperative, operative, and postoperative elements have been recognized as essential to providing the standard of care for patients with pancreatic cancer.[3,4] All centers, regardless of volume, must implement these elements and track their outcomes to ensure they are meeting the standard.

This article discusses the implementation of these key elements of pancreatic cancer care during the development of a successful pancreatic surgery program at a large tertiary care community hospital. Carolinas Medical Center (CMC) has rapidly transitioned from a low- to a high-volume center for pancreatic cancer surgery since the inception of the hepatopancreatobiliary (HPB) surgery program in October 2006. This rapid emergence of a high-volume pancreatic care center in an area where patients may not have been referred for surgery previously, had their surgery at low-volume community hospitals in the area, or were referred elsewhere for surgery has had a substantial effect on pancreatic cancer care in the surrounding community and central and western North Carolina.

CHANGING DEMOGRAPHICS AFTER THE INTRODUCTION OF A NEW REGIONAL HPB REFERRAL CENTER

The CMC HPB program was initiated in late 2006 to respond to a need for specialized HPB surgery in central and western North Carolina. CMC, a large tertiary care community teaching hospital, subsequently transitioned from a low- to a high-volume center in late 2006. To investigate the impact of this new referral center, the North Carolina Hospital Discharge Database (Thomson Reuters, Fiscal Years 2004–2009) was queried for all patients undergoing resection for pancreatic cancer from 2004 to 2009. Hospitals were then divided into volume categories based upon the total number of pancreaticoduodenectomy operations performed for cancer per year, with low-volume consisting of <5 PD/year, mid- volume consisting of 5–9 PD/year, and high-volume consisting of 10 or more PD/year. The annual distribution of cases to low-, mid-, and high-volume centers over this time span reflects a consistent trend toward regionalization to high-volume centers in North Carolina (**Fig. 1**A, B) and toward large centers that have more resources available, such as the ability to support

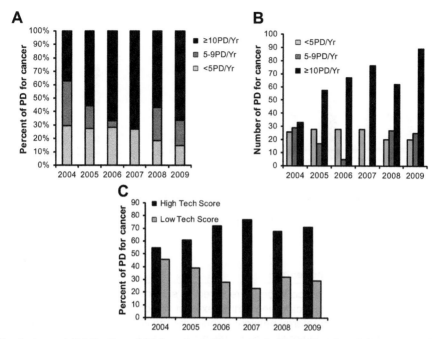

Fig. 1. Annual distribution of PD for pancreatic cancer in North Carolina. (*A*) Percentage of total number of PDs performed in North Carolina for low-, medium-, and high-volume hospitals. (*B*) Distribution to hospitals with low- (<5 PDs per year), medium- (5–9 PDs per year), or high-volume (≥10 PDs per year). (*C*) Distribution of PD to hospitals categorized as having a high or low technology score, as defined by ability to support solid organ transplant and open heart surgery programs.

solid organ transplant and open heart surgery programs (**Fig. 1**C).[31] The designation of academic or community hospital is less important than possessing the appropriate resources to perform complex operations such as pancreatic resection.

These data suggest an increase in regionalization to centers that specialize in pancreatic cancer care in North Carolina since 2004. A concomitant push toward regionalization has undoubtedly occurred nationwide, and these statewide data likely reflect this trend; however, these data also support the idea that being properly equipped to deliver high-quality pancreatic cancer care is the most important factor in determining referral patterns. The CMC HPB program was instituted in the middle of this timeframe, and has undoubtedly contributed to this increase in regionalization.

Growth of the CMC HPB program since October 2006 has been exponential. New patient office visits and consultations for all HPB diseases have increased from 244 in 2007 to 460 in 2009, an increase of 189% (**Fig. 2**A). Case-specific volume has also increased, with 16 PDs performed in 2007 for all causes, and 72 performed for all causes in 2009, an increase of 450% (**Fig. 2**B).

KEY COMPONENTS OF A PANCREATIC CANCER CARE PROGRAM

Multiple components are essential for the delivery of high-quality pancreatic cancer care, regardless of the hospital setting in which it is delivered. This article describes these components and their integration into the CMC program as it was developed.

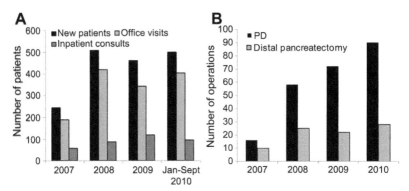

Fig. 2. CMC HPB growth since the program began in October 2006. (*A*) Annual number of new patients seen in the office and inpatient setting. (*B*) Annual number of PDs and distal pancreatectomies performed at CMC. (These data were compiled from internal CMC sources.)

Essential Hospital Components

Hospital location is a key component required to support a pancreatic cancer care program. In short, a significant need must exist in the community, and the hospital must establish a strong referral network throughout the community. In a recent analysis of all patients with potentially resectable stage I pancreatic cancer in the National Cancer Database from 1995 to 2004, only 28.6% underwent surgery. Of the remaining 71.4%, a disturbingly high percentage (38.2%) were never offered surgery, and another 13.5% had no recorded reason for not undergoing surgery.[32] This underuse of the only curative option for patients with stage I pancreatic cancer suggests a pessimistic view of the outcomes of pancreatic resection and the survival of pancreatic cancer patients in general.

A major service to the community is simply spreading the word to the treating physicians in the region that a safe and effective pancreatic surgery option is available to their patients with pancreatic cancer. Equally important is the need to update physicians outside the oncologic community regarding the quickly evolving treatment algorithms for pancreatic cancer. For example, the cancer that was considered unresectable in the past may be amenable to neoadjuvant chemoradiation followed by resection today,[33] and the dreaded CT scan showing portal vein involvement is no longer an absolute contraindication to resection.[34] Given these advances, even experienced surgeons in centers capable of supporting routine pancreatic resection should, when treating high-risk patients with difficult anatomy, consider referral for a second opinion rather than deeming these patients inoperable. Establishing a strong referral and education network in the community is key to maximizing the use of surgical resection in patients who deserve that option.

The CMC HPB program was established in a region where patients were either not being referred for pancreatic resection, being referred and deemed unresectable, or being referred elsewhere for pancreatic resection. The Carolinas Healthcare System includes more than 30 hospitals in North and South Carolina, thus facilitating the process of implementing a referral mechanism within the system.

The ability of the staff at a hospital to recognize and respond appropriately to a postoperative complication is a key aspect of patient care after pancreatic resection. In reviewing the Nationwide Inpatient Sample for pancreatic resections from 2000 to 2006, five hospital characteristics known to be associated with improved outcomes were tested for an effect on "failure to rescue," defined as inability to prevent death after a major complication. These variables included teaching status, size greater than 200 beds, average census more than 50% full, increased nurse-to-patient ratio, and high hospital technology scores (defined as the ability to support an open heart and solid organ transplant service). All of the variables tested were associated with improved ability to prevent death from a major postoperative complication, supporting the idea that certain elements of hospital structure and process are essential to ensuring excellent outcomes after pancreatic surgery.[31] CMC is a 1000-bed tertiary care teaching hospital that supports busy cardiac surgery and solid organ transplant programs, and has a general surgery residency program and multiple surgical fellowships.

Essential Components of an HPB Service

One of the major contributors to the improved outcomes seen at high-volume hospitals for select technically complex operations is the individual surgeon volume at these high-volume hospitals,[35,36] which appears to be particularly important for pancreaticoduodenectomy.[30,36,37] Birkmeyer and colleagues[35] analyzed the Medical Provider Analysis and Review (MEDPAR) files for all Medicare patients undergoing 1 of 14 major cardiovascular or cancer operations in 1998 and 1999. For pancreatic resection for cancer, they showed that 54% of the decrease in hospital mortality seen at high-volume centers could be attributed to surgeon volume. Similarly, in a risk-adjusted analysis of the Nationwide Inpatient Sample for all pancreatic resections performed from 1998 to 2005, in which surgeon and hospital identifiers were recorded, high-volume surgeons were associated with an even lower risk of mortality than high-volume hospitals.[37] Inpatient mortality after pancreatic resection seems to be the most surgeon-dependent compared with other complex hepatobiliary operations. This finding is reflected in an analysis of the State Inpatient Databases for three states that record both hospital- and surgeon-specific data. In this analysis, high-volume centers had lower mortality than low-volume centers for all complex HPB operations; however, for PD this difference was largely attributable to high-volume surgeons, pointing toward the high operative expertise required for this specific procedure.[30]

Because a notable learning curve exists for performance of pancreatic resections, surgeons who perform pancreatic resections must have adequate experience.[38,39] In a review of outcomes after pancreatic resection at one high-volume cancer center spanning 15 years, a comparison of three surgeons' first versus second 60 PDs showed that increased experience resulted in lower margin positivity, higher lymph node yield, shorter length of stay, shorter operative times, and less blood loss.[38] Similarly, in an analysis of PDs performed at another high-volume referral center for pancreatic cancer care, surgeons who had performed more than 50 PDs in their career had significantly lower morbidity, shorter operative times, and less blood loss than less experienced surgeons, despite performing significantly more complex vascular resections in conjunction with the PD.[39] For the generation of surgeons emerging from surgical residency today, this means that additional fellowship training is essential to ensure adequate outcomes. The establishment of an HPB program at CMC was predicated on recruiting experienced board-certified fellowship-trained HPB surgeons, and the dedication to this advanced training is evidenced by the establishment of an accredited HPB fellowship program.

Regarding the structure of an HPB service, the authors have found that the establishment of a separate HPB call schedule and service, including an HPB clinical fellow and residents, dedicated mid-level providers, and dedicated operating room and clinical nursing staff, is highly beneficial in the coordination of care for these patients. In caring for a predominantly older population undergoing major pancreatic resection, it is essential to maximize continuity of care and minimize the "hand-offs" and "cross-coverage" that can lead to communication error, particularly in the current era of residency work-hour restrictions.

Essential Components of Nonsurgical Departments

As important as the surgeons and HPB service are, delivery of quality care to patients with pancreatic cancer involves much more than the surgical team. Recruiting and establishing HPB expertise across departments is absolutely essential.

Strong medical and radiation oncology programs should be in place for optimal preoperative and postoperative pancreatic cancer treatment programs. Adjuvant gemcitabine-based chemotherapy is now well-known to improve survival after pancreatic cancer resection and is considered standard of care.[40–42] The evidence for adjuvant radiation therapy is less well established; however, its use in combination with gemcitabine-based chemotherapy in the neoadjuvant setting may decrease margin-positive resection and improve survival.[43–45] This use may be particularly applicable in the "borderline" resectable patient in whom the extent of local disease is formidable.[34] Keeping in mind the fact that 70% to 80% of patients with pancreatic cancer will not be candidates for resection, an experienced and capable medical oncology program must also be in place to offer the best available treatment for these patients. A team approach to pancreatic cancer resection, implementing all three forms of therapy as indicated, is critical to meeting the standard of care for pancreas surgery.

The gastrointestinal medicine department at a pancreatic cancer care center should incorporate expertise in endoscopic ultrasound (EUS) and endoscopic retrograde cholangiopancreatography (ERCP). Like other ultrasound procedures, performance of EUS is heavily operator-dependent, and requires advanced training beyond a gastrointestinal fellowship and a minimum number of proctored cases to obtain certification.[46] EUS has a reported T-stage accuracy of 78% to 94% and N-stage accuracy of 64% to 82% across several series,[47] and is more sensitive for detecting small tumors (<2 cm in diameter) and suspicious lymph nodes than both CT and MRI.[46,48] EUS also offers the advantage of allowing guided fine needle aspiration (FNA) of pancreatic masses and adjacent lymph nodes, with a reported diagnostic accuracy of 72% for pancreatic cancer.[46] However, in addition to endoscopist expertise, pathologist experience in evaluating cytologic specimens from EUS-guided FNA is required to reach the full diagnostic potential. EUS-guided FNA is more specific (98%) than sensitive (85%), meaning that a negative result does not definitively rule out cancer. Thus, its use is particularly advantageous in patients who have suspicious lymph nodes outside of the resection field or who have a low suspicion of pancreatic cancer, thus decreasing the possibility of performing an unnecessary resection.[48]

Given these advantages in diagnosis and patient selection, the institution of an EUS program is an indispensible part of any pancreatic cancer care program. After the HPB program was established at CMC, an EUS program was started in the fall of 2007. The annual volume has continued to expand, with EUS performed in 1730 patients in 3 years. More than 60% of these patients were being evaluated for HPB-related disease.

Expertise in ERCP also requires advanced training beyond a gastrointestinal fellowship. Expertise in ERCP and common bile duct (CBD) stent placement should be readily available for the preoperative evaluation of many patients with pancreatic cancer and biliary obstruction. Although previously, CBD stents were routinely placed in all of these patients, its indication for biliary obstruction has narrowed recently. A recent review showed that stent-related complications led to a significant delay in resection and an increased postoperative infection rate in patients who underwent preoperative biliary drainage, thus challenging the efficacy of routine preoperative drainage.[49] However, biliary drainage in symptomatic potentially resectable patients, and those with obstruction secondary to unresectable cancer, remains a mainstay in the complete approach to pancreatic cancer care.

The radiology department is an integral part of a pancreatic cancer care program. The resources and expertise to perform and interpret state-of-the-art pancreatic imaging should be available. Pancreatic protocol CT scan, with arterial and delayed portal venous phases, is the authors' preferred imaging modality for pancreatic tumors, and is highly accurate for detecting tumors as small as 1.5 to 2 cm.[50] Assessment of the superior mesenteric vein (SMV), portal vein (PV), superior mesenteric artery (SMA), and hepatic artery for vessel invasion, and the liver and lungs for distant metastatic disease, makes pancreatic protocol CT the ideal modality for assessment of resectability.[51] The combination of pancreatic protocol CT and EUS provides the best imaging framework for pancreatic cancer staging. Other imaging modalities, such as MRI, magnetic resonance cholangiopancreatography (MRCP), and positron emission tomography/CT (PET/CT) have a role to play in select patients, and should be readily available, although they are not currently routinely used.[51]

Even at centers with excellent pancreatic surgeons, complications such as intra-abdominal abscess formation and anastomotic leaks undoubtedly will occur after pancreatic surgery, and therefore these complications must be recognized and managed efficiently. A skilled on-site interventional radiology department is essential to help treat these patients after a complication. Postoperative abscess drainage, percutaneous transhepatic cholangiography/biliary drainage, and arterial embolization are common minimally invasive methods that can prevent the morbidity of a second trip to the operating room for these patients.[52]

The anesthesia department plays a very important role in the perioperative care of patients undergoing pancreatic resection. Expertise in managing the intraoperative volume status and regional pain control for these patients is critical.[53] The authors have found that working with a dedicated group of anesthesia staff and Certified Registered Nurse Anesthetists familiar with the requirements of an HPB operation is very beneficial. Similarly, a critical care team familiar with management issues of these patients, who are often older and frail, after pancreatic resection is essential to ensure optimal outcomes. Twenty-four-hour intensive care unit staffing by an intensivist is now considered standard of care.[54]

Finally, the pathology department is also important in the team approach to pancreatic cancer resection. Expertise in interpreting and reporting cytology from EUS-guided FNA and surgical resection specimens is essential. The PD specimen should be inked and sectioned to evaluate margins of transection (duodenum, bile duct, pancreatic neck, jejunum), radial retroperitoneal margins, and the margin between the uncinate process and the SMA.[34] This thorough evaluation requires coordination between the pathologist and the surgeon. The authors have found it highly beneficial to personally take the specimen to the pathology laboratory and mark it together with the pathologist. The tumor grade, number of positive lymph nodes, and total number of lymph nodes resected should be routinely reported in a consistent manner.[3]

Performing pancreatic cancer resections in a hospital that is dedicated to broad cancer care offers other benefits that cannot be overlooked. Patients who have undergone pancreatic resection often require specific diet and medication adjustments for

| **Box 1** |
| **Preoperative, operative, and postoperative variables required for tracking outcomes in pancreatic surgery** |

Preoperative

Medical history

    Risk factors and comorbid diseases

Presentation

    Emergent/urgent/elective

Tumor markers

    CA 19.9

Cross-sectional imaging

    Location, size, and character of mass

    Vascular involvement

    Suspicious nodal disease

    Metastatic disease

Endoscopic ultrasound

    Location, size, and character of mass

    Vascular involvement

    Suspicious nodal disease

    FNA cytology results

Endoscopic retrograde cholangiopancreatography

    Presence of a stricture or mass

    Brushing cytology results

    Stent placement

Clinical Stage

    TNM stage by current American Joint Committee on Cancer (AJCC) guidelines

Assessment of resectability

    Resectable/borderline/locally advanced

Neoadjuvant treatment

    Type and duration of treatment

Operative

Operating room

    Results of exploration for metastatic disease

    Type of resection performed

    Method of reconstruction

    Vascular resection/reconstruction

    Extent of lymphadenectomy

    Skeletonization of superior mesenteric artery

    Frozen section margin results

    Estimated blood loss

    Operative time

Pathology

    Tumor size, location, and grade

    TMN stage by current AJCC guidelines

    Number of lymph nodes resected

    Treatment effect

    Lymphovascular/perineural invasion

    Margin status

Postoperative

Morbidity and mortality

    Pancreatic fistula rate by International study group of pancreatic fistula definition

    Postoperative complication rate and type

    30- and 90-day mortality rate

Adjuvant treatment

    Type and duration of treatment

Recurrence

    Timing and location of recurrence

Survival

    2- and 5-year survival

issues such as delayed gastric emptying and pancreatic insufficiency. Having a dedicated nutritionist program to help these patients with these difficult transitions is very helpful. Providing patient advocates who can help these patients navigate the complex cancer care network and explain treatment options also benefits patients tremendously.

Coordination of a detailed plan of action for these patients is a difficult task that mandates weekly multidisciplinary conferences incorporating all of the specialties mentioned earlier. The authors have found it beneficial to establish weekly multidisciplinary HPB and gastrointestinal tumor planning conferences, which are video-linked to multiple hospitals within the Carolinas Healthcare System.

Operative Technique

The technique of performing a PD has long been debated, and currently no consensus exists on the superiority of pylorus-preserving versus standard resection or type of pancreaticojejunostomy.[55,56] Many centers have published excellent results using the technique that they have perfected; however, probably more important than the actual technique is that the surgeon performing the operation be facile and meticulous with the selected method. For example, the surgeons at CMC have found that a pylorus-preserving PD with a duct-to-mucosal anastomosis with the addition of a buttress of vascularized round ligament minimizes the postoperative pancreatic leak rate.[57] Vastly more important than the choice of resection and reconstruction technique is the adherence to and documentation of standard oncologic principles, including thorough evaluation of resectability, skeletonization of the SMA, standard lymphadenectomy, and a coordinated approach with the pathologist for evaluation of margins.[58]

Unfortunately, even when a standard technique is optimized and sound principles of resection are in place, not all pancreatic resections will fit the mold for a routine PD. When offering resection to patients with borderline resectable tumors, the ability to incorporate vascular resection and reconstruction without compounding morbidity is essential.[34] Despite modern imaging, the surgeon often does not know with absolute certainty whether vascular resection will be required before beginning the operation. Occasionally, vascular invasion is not apparent until after the surgeon is committed to resection. If these procedures are beyond the scope of the program at a given center, patients with borderline resectable tumors should be offered referral for evaluation at a center with these capabilities before exploration.

Tracking of Patient Outcomes

With the current focus in the medical community and the general public on the issues of patient safety and surgical outcomes, the hospital and surgeon performing pancreatic surgery must track and record their experience, including multiple preoperative, operative, and postoperative variables (**Box 1**). Often these data are collected and stored by the surgeon or department in personal or departmental databases, with obvious variation in the breadth of the data points collected. Any concerted effort to track and understand surgical outcomes should be applauded; however, a centralized uniform method for collecting and reporting these data will become essential as the requirements for strict surgical quality control continue to expand.

Perioperative data should include enough preoperative variables to adequately risk-adjust for the severity of illness and case complexity. Therefore, centers that treat the most complex cases in the most high-risk patients are not penalized for potentially higher morbidity and mortality rates. In other words, apples can be compared with apples. Although this sounds like a tall order for any institution, the framework for this system has been laid out by the Veterans Affairs (VA) National Surgical Quality Improvement Program (NSQIP) in collaboration with the American College of Surgeons (ACS).[59] The NSQIP was implemented in all VA hospitals in the 1990s in response to a perceived inferiority of surgical care at VA hospitals, and resulted in unprecedented improvements in postoperative morbidity and mortality.[60] This framework has been adapted to the private sector with similar results, and could be applied successfully to HPB procedures.[61]

The recording and reporting of this information in a risk-adjusted manner is in the best interest of the patient, because it allows them to make an educated decision when choosing a center or surgeon for pancreatic resection. It is also in the best interest of the hospital and surgeon to understand the results of their work, because examining one's own results undoubtedly leads to improvement. Furthermore, the strengths and limitations of one's own hospital system are important to know, as is recognizing which high-risk patients or procedures will require resources that are outside the scope of the current hospital structure, and therefore should be referred to a center with an established system in that area.[62] Until a risk-adjusted national HPB database is available, the HPB program at CMC is currently tracking patient outcomes internally and is establishing a Web-based secure HPB database to meet this immediate requirement (Research Electronic Data Capture [REDCap]).[63]

Participation in Institutional and National Clinical Trials

Treatment of pancreatic cancer has advanced significantly in the past 30 years. These advances are the result of the hard work and collaboration required to plan and implement well-designed institutional and national clinical research protocols. It is imperative that hospitals and surgeons who elect to participate in the care of patients with pancreatic cancer also participate in the research that moves this field forward. The surgeon also has much to offer the basic scientist, such as access to human disease and a clinical perspective; therefore, collaborative efforts in basic science should be sought.

SUMMARY

Pancreatic resection can be performed safely in the community-based hospital setting only when appropriate systems are in place for patient selection and preoperative, operative, and postoperative care. Pancreatic surgery cannot be performed optimally without considerable investment in and coordination of multiple departments. Delivery of high-quality pancreatic cancer care demands a rigorous assessment of the hospital structure and the processes through which this care is delivered; however, when a hospital makes the considerable effort to establish the necessary systems required for delivery of quality pancreatic cancer care, the community and hospital will benefit substantially.

REFERENCES

1. Jemal A, Siegel R, Xu J, et al. Cancer statistics, 2010. CA Cancer J Clin 2010; 60(5):277–300.
2. Riall TS, Nealon WH, Goodwin JS, et al. Pancreatic cancer in the general population: improvements in survival over the last decade. J Gastrointest Surg 2006; 10(9):1212–23 [discussion: 1223–4].
3. Bilimoria KY, Bentrem DJ, Lillemoe KD, et al. Assessment of pancreatic cancer care in the United States based on formally developed quality indicators. J Natl Cancer Inst 2009;101(12):848–59.
4. Raval MV, Bilimoria KY, Talamonti MS. Quality improvement for pancreatic cancer care: is regionalization a feasible and effective mechanism? Surg Oncol Clin N Am 2010;19(2):371–90.
5. Khuri SF, Henderson WG. The case against volume as a measure of quality of surgical care. World J Surg 2005;29(10):1222–9.
6. Birkmeyer JD, Dimick JB. Understanding and reducing variation in surgical mortality. Annu Rev Med 2009;60:405–15.
7. Balzano G, Zerbi A, Capretti G, et al. Effect of hospital volume on outcome of pancreaticoduodenectomy in Italy. Br J Surg 2008;95(3):357–62.
8. Birkmeyer JD, Finlayson SR, Tosteson AN, et al. Effect of hospital volume on in-hospital mortality with pancreaticoduodenectomy. Surgery 1999;125(3):250–6.
9. Birkmeyer JD, Warshaw AL, Finlayson SR, et al. Relationship between hospital volume and late survival after pancreaticoduodenectomy. Surgery 1999;126(2): 178–83.
10. Fong Y, Gonen M, Rubin D, et al. Long-term survival is superior after resection for cancer in high-volume centers. Ann Surg 2005;242(4):540–4 [discussion: 544–7].
11. McPhee JT, Hill JS, Whalen GF, et al. Perioperative mortality for pancreatectomy: a national perspective. Ann Surg 2007;246(2):246–53.
12. Topal B, Van de Sande S, Fieuws S, et al. Effect of centralization of pancreaticoduodenectomy on nationwide hospital mortality and length of stay. Br J Surg 2007;94(11):1377–81.
13. van Heek NT, Kuhlmann KF, Scholten RJ, et al. Hospital volume and mortality after pancreatic resection: a systematic review and an evaluation of intervention in the Netherlands. Ann Surg 2005;242(6):781–8 [discussion: 788–90].

14. Glasgow RE, Mulvihill SJ. Hospital volume influences outcome in patients under-going pancreatic resection for cancer. West J Med 1996;165(5):294–300.

15. Sosa JA, Bowman HM, Gordon TA, et al. Importance of hospital volume in the overall management of pancreatic cancer. Ann Surg 1998;228(3):429–38.

16. Lieberman MD, Kilburn H, Lindsey M, et al. Relation of perioperative deaths to hospital volume among patients undergoing pancreatic resection for malignancy. Ann Surg 1995;222(5):638–45.

17. Birkmeyer JD, Siewers AE, Marth NJ, et al. Regionalization of high-risk surgery and implications for patient travel times. JAMA 2003;290(20):2703–8.

18. Finlayson SR, Birkmeyer JD, Tosteson AN, et al. Patient preferences for location of care: implications for regionalization. Med Care 1999;37(2):204–9.

19. Dimick JB, Finlayson SR. Rural hospitals and volume standards in surgery. Surgery 2006;140(3):367–71.

20. Riall TS, Eschbach KA, Townsend CM Jr, et al. Trends and disparities in region-alization of pancreatic resection. J Gastrointest Surg 2007;11(10):1242–51 [discussion: 1251–2].

21. Gordon TA, Bowman HM, Tielsch JM, et al. Statewide regionalization of pancrea-ticoduodenectomy and its effect on in-hospital mortality. Ann Surg 1998;228(1):71–8.

22. Nienhuijs SW, Rutten HJ, Luiten EJ, et al. Reduction of in-hospital mortality following regionalisation of pancreatic surgery in the south-east of the Netherlands. Eur J Surg Oncol 2010;36(7):652–6.

23. Cunningham JD, O'Donnell N, Starker P. Surgical outcomes following pancreatic resection at a low-volume community hospital: do all patients need to be sent to a regional cancer center? Am J Surg 2009;198(2):227–30.

24. Metreveli RE, Sahm K, Abdel-Misih R, et al. Major pancreatic resections for sus-pected cancer in a community-based teaching hospital: lessons learned. J Surg Oncol 2007;95(3):201–6.

25. Peros G, Giannopoulos GA, Christodoulou S, et al. Good results after major pancreatic resections in a middle-volume center. Pancreas 2010;39(3):411–4.

26. Chew DK, Attiyeh FF. Experience with the Whipple procedure (pancreaticoduo-denectomy) in a university-affiliated community hospital. Am J Surg 1997;174(3):312–5.

27. Cocieru A, Saldinger PF. HPB surgery can be safely performed in a community teaching hospital. J Gastrointest Surg 2010;14(11):1853–7.

28. Joseph B, Morton JM, Hernandez-Boussard T, et al. Relationship between hospital volume, system clinical resources, and mortality in pancreatic resection. J Am Coll Surg 2009;208(4):520–7.

29. Teh SH, Diggs BS, Deveney CW, et al. Patient and hospital characteristics on the variance of perioperative outcomes for pancreatic resection in the United States: a plea for outcome-based and not volume-based referral guidelines. Arch Surg 2009;144(8):713–21.

30. Nathan H, Cameron JL, Choti MA, et al. The volume-outcomes effect in hepato-pancreato-biliary surgery: hospital versus surgeon contributions and specificity of the relationship. J Am Coll Surg 2009;208(4):528–38.

31. Ghaferi AA, Osborne NH, Birkmeyer JD, et al. Hospital characteristics associated with failure to rescue from complications after pancreatectomy. J Am Coll Surg 2010;211(3):325–30.

32. Bilimoria KY, Bentrem DJ, Ko CY, et al. National failure to operate on early stage pancreatic cancer. Ann Surg 2007;246(2):173–80.

33. Abrams RA, Lowy AM, O'Reilly EM, et al. Combined modality treatment of resectable and borderline resectable pancreas cancer: expert consensus statement. Ann Surg Oncol 2009;16(7):1751–6.
34. Evans DB, Farnell MB, Lillemoe KD, et al. Surgical treatment of resectable and borderline resectable pancreas cancer: expert consensus statement. Ann Surg Oncol 2009;16(7):1736–44.
35. Birkmeyer JD, Stukel TA, Siewers AE, et al. Surgeon volume and operative mortality in the United States. N Engl J Med 2003;349(22):2117–27.
36. Kennedy TJ, Cassera MA, Wolf R, et al. Surgeon volume versus morbidity and cost in patients undergoing pancreaticoduodenectomy in an academic community medical center. J Gastrointest Surg 2010;14(12):1990–6.
37. Eppsteiner RW, Csikesz NG, McPhee JT, et al. Surgeon volume impacts hospital mortality for pancreatic resection. Ann Surg 2009;249(4):635–40.
38. Tseng JF, Pisters PW, Lee JE, et al. The learning curve in pancreatic surgery. Surgery 2007;141(5):694–701.
39. Schmidt CM, Turrini O, Parikh P, et al. Effect of hospital volume, surgeon experience, and surgeon volume on patient outcomes after pancreaticoduodenectomy: a single-institution experience. Arch Surg 2010;145(7):634–40.
40. Oettle H, Post S, Neuhaus P, et al. Adjuvant chemotherapy with gemcitabine vs observation in patients undergoing curative-intent resection of pancreatic cancer: a randomized controlled trial. JAMA 2007;297(3):267–77.
41. Neoptolemos JP, Stocken DD, Bassi C, et al. Adjuvant chemotherapy with fluorouracil plus folinic acid vs gemcitabine following pancreatic cancer resection: a randomized controlled trial. JAMA 2010;304(10):1073–81.
42. Ueno H, Kosuge T, Matsuyama Y, et al. A randomised phase III trial comparing gemcitabine with surgery-only in patients with resected pancreatic cancer: Japanese Study Group of Adjuvant Therapy for Pancreatic Cancer. Br J Cancer 2009; 101(6):908–15.
43. Klinkenbijl JH, Jeekel J, Sahmoud T, et al. Adjuvant radiotherapy and 5-fluorouracil after curative resection of cancer of the pancreas and periampullary region: phase III trial of the EORTC gastrointestinal tract cancer cooperative group. Ann Surg 1999;230(6):776–82 [discussion: 782–4].
44. Nugent FW, Stuart K. Adjuvant and neoadjuvant therapy in curable pancreatic cancer. Surg Clin North Am 2010;90(2):323–39.
45. Evans DB, Varadhachary GR, Crane CH, et al. Preoperative gemcitabine-based chemoradiation for patients with resectable adenocarcinoma of the pancreatic head. J Clin Oncol 2008;26(21):3496–502.
46. Owens DJ, Savides TJ. Endoscopic ultrasound staging and novel therapeutics for pancreatic cancer. Surg Oncol Clin N Am 2010;19(2):255–66.
47. Hunt GC, Faigel DO. Assessment of EUS for diagnosing, staging, and determining resectability of pancreatic cancer: a review. Gastrointest Endosc 2002; 55(2):232–7.
48. Varadarajulu S, Eloubeidi MA. The role of endoscopic ultrasonography in the evaluation of pancreatico-biliary cancer. Surg Clin North Am 2010;90(2):251–63.
49. Mezhir JJ, Brennan MF, Baser RE, et al. A matched case-control study of preoperative biliary drainage in patients with pancreatic adenocarcinoma: routine drainage is not justified. J Gastrointest Surg 2009;13(12):2163–9.
50. Bronstein YL, Loyer EM, Kaur H, et al. Detection of small pancreatic tumors with multiphasic helical CT. AJR Am J Roentgenol 2004;182(3):619–23.
51. Kinney T. Evidence-based imaging of pancreatic malignancies. Surg Clin North Am 2010;90(2):235–49.

52. Sohn TA, Yeo CJ, Cameron JL, et al. Pancreaticoduodenectomy: role of interventional radiologists in managing patients and complications. J Gastrointest Surg 2003;7(2):209–19.

53. Marandola M, Cilli T, Alessandri F, et al. Perioperative management in patients undergoing pancreatic surgery: the anesthesiologist's point of view. Transplant Proc 2008;40(4):1195–9.

54. Pronovost PJ, Angus DC, Dorman T, et al. Physician staffing patterns and clinical outcomes in critically ill patients: a systematic review. JAMA 2002;288(17):2151–62.

55. Diener MK, Knaebel HP, Heukaufer C, et al. A systematic review and meta-analysis of pylorus-preserving versus classical pancreaticoduodenectomy for surgical treatment of periampullary and pancreatic carcinoma. Ann Surg 2007; 245(2):187–200.

56. Kennedy EP, Brumbaugh J, Yeo CJ. Reconstruction following the pylorus preserving Whipple resection: PJ, HJ, and DJ. J Gastrointest Surg 2010;14(2): 408–15.

57. Iannitti DA, Coburn NG, Somberg J, et al. Use of the round ligament of the liver to decrease pancreatic fistulas: a novel technique. J Am Coll Surg 2006;203(6): 857–64.

58. Katz MH, Merchant NB, Brower S, et al. Standardization of Surgical and pathologic variables is needed in multicenter trials of adjuvant therapy for pancreatic cancer: results from the ACOSOG Z5031 trial. Ann Surg Oncol 2010;18(2): 337–44.

59. Khuri SF, Henderson WG, Daley J, et al. Successful implementation of the Department of Veterans Affairs' National Surgical Quality Improvement Program in the private sector: the patient safety in surgery study. Ann Surg 2008;248(2):329–36.

60. Khuri SF, Henderson WG, Daley J, et al. The patient safety in surgery study: background, study design, and patient populations. J Am Coll Surg 2007;204(6): 1089–102.

61. Pitt HA, Kilbane M, Strasberg SM, et al. ACS-NSQIP has the potential to create an HPB-NSQIP option. HPB (Oxford) 2009;11(5):405–13.

62. Bilimoria KY, Bentrem DJ, Talamonti MS, et al. Risk-based selective referral for cancer surgery: a potential strategy to improve perioperative outcomes. Ann Surg 2010;251(4):708–16.

63. Harris PA, Taylor R, Thielke R, et al. Research electronic data capture (REDCap) - A metadata-driven methodology and workflow process for providing translational research informatics support. J Biomed Inform 2009;42(2):377–81.

Maximizing Rectal Cancer Results: TEM and TATA Techniques to Expand Sphincter Preservation

John H. Marks, MD[a,b,c,d,*], Joseph L. Frenkel, MD[e],
Anthony P. D'Andrea, MS[f], Chistopher E. Greenleaf, MD[g]

KEYWORDS

- Rectal cancer • Laparoscopy
- Transanal endoscopic microsurgery • Neoadjuvant radiation
- Low anterior resection

Colorectal cancer remains the number one abdominal-visceral cancer afflicting both men and women in America. With more than 104,000 new cases diagnosed each year, the incidence of colorectal cancer, while decreasing slightly over the past decade, still remains terribly high.[1,2] The fact that this cancer is preceded by a premalignant condition of a polyp that can be eradicated by colonoscopy and polypectomy makes this high incidence all the more frustrating. There are a multitude of reasons for avoidance of screening; however, the greatest fraction seems to be the patients'

The authors have nothing to disclose.

[a] Lankenau Hospital Colorectal Center, 100 East Lancaster Avenue, Medical Office Building West, Suite 330, Wynnewood, PA 19096, USA

[b] Main Line Health Systems, 100 East Lancaster Avenue, Wynnewood, PA 19096, USA

[c] Division of Colorectal Surgery, Lankenau Hospital, 100 East Lancaster Avenue, Lankenau Medical Office Building West, Suite 330, Wynnewood, PA 19096, USA

[d] Lankenau Institute of Medical Research, 100 East Lancaster Avenue, Wynnewood, PA 19096, USA

[e] Minimally Invasive Colorectal Surgery and Rectal Cancer Fellow, Division of Colorectal Surgery, Lankenau Hospital, 100 East Lancaster Avenue, Lankenau Medical Office Building West, Suite 330, Wynnewood, PA 19096, USA

[f] Division of Colorectal Surgery, Marks Colorectal Surgical Foundation, Lankenau Hospital, 100 East Lancaster Avenue, Lankenau Medical Office Building West, Suite 330, Wynnewood, PA 19096, USA

[g] Division of Graduate Medical Education, Lankenau Hospital, 100 East Lancaster Avenue, Wynnewood, PA 19096, USA

* Corresponding author. Division of Colorectal Surgery, Lankenau Hospital, 100 East Lancaster Avenue, Lankenau Medical Office Building West, Suite 330, Wynnewood, PA 19096.
E-mail address: MarksJ@mlhs.org

reluctance to undergo the discomfort of bowel preparation as well as fears of the need for a permanent colostomy. Of all colorectal cancers diagnosed annually in the United States, 40,000 of these are rectal cancers. It is in this region that concerns for ultimate cure are higher, prevention of recurrence is more challenging, and the risk of a permanent colostomy is a very real possibility.

The current TNM classification system has evolved as a very useful way of discussing all cancers (**Table 1**). Historically, rectal cancer was discussed in Duke's stage A, B, C, and D, which correlates with TNM Stage 1, 2, 3, and 4. For the purpose of this article as well as any discussion of rectal cancer in the 21st century, the TNM classification system should be used (**Table 2**). In terms of discussing matters, Stage 1 disease is node-negative rectal cancer confined to the rectal wall. Stage 2 disease is node-negative rectal cancer that has extended through the rectal wall. Stage 3 disease is any T stage with node positivity. Stage 4 disease is any T or N stage with metastatic disease present. It is essential to emphasize and review this so we can have a common lexicon to discuss cancer therapy.

A multitude of issues exists regarding the treatment of patients with rectal cancer. Questions surround both the surgical management as well as the use of adjuvant therapy, and they impound in the literature. Concerns are always focused first and foremost on how various treatment strategies affect recurrence rates and survival; however, in patients with rectal cancer quality of life and body image are closely intertwined with these disease-specific outcomes. Because of this, the major issue of abdominoperineal resection (APR) rates with resulting permanent colostomy comes into focus.

Table 1	
TNM staging for colorectal cancer	
T Staging	
T1	Lamina propria or submucosa or ≤2 cm
T1a	<1 cm
T1b	1 to 2 cm
T2	Muscularis propria or >2 cm
T3	Subserosa or pericolorectal tissues
T4	Tumor directly invades other organs or structures and/or perforates visceral peritoneum
T4a	Perforates visceral peritoneum
T4b	Directly invades other organ or structures
N Staging	
N1	Metastasis in 1 to 3 regional lymph nodes
N1a	1 node
N1b	2–3 nodes
N1c	Satellites in subserosa *without* regional nodes
N2	Metastasis in 4 or more regional lymph nodes
N2a	4–6 nodes
N2b	7 or more nodes
M Staging (Distant Metastasis)	
M1a	One organ
M1b	>one organ or peritoneum

Data from Sobin LH, Gospodarowicz MK, Wittekind C, editors. International Union Against Cancer. TNM classification of malignant tumours. 7th edition. Chichester (UK): Wiley-Blackwell; 2009.

Table 2 TNM classification system		
TNM Stage		**Duke's Stage**
I	T1–2, N0, M0	A
II	T3–4, N0, M0	B
III	T any, N1–3, M0	C
IV	T any, N any, M1	D

Data from Sobin LH, Gospodarowicz MK, Wittekind C, editors. International Union Against Cancer. TNM Classification of malignant tumours. 7th edition. Chichester (UK): Wiley-Blackwell; 2009.

To achieve the goals of both optimal oncologic outcomes with a high quality of life, multimodal therapy has come to the forefront of rectal cancer management. Questions regarding both chemotherapy and radiation are multiple. The most basic question, however, is whether adjuvant treatment should be given preoperatively or postoperatively.

From a surgical standpoint, technical issues involve the necessity of performing a total mesorectal excision as well as what the role of local excision may be. To add even further complexity to this, we must consider whether these surgical options may be modified based on the response of the rectal cancer to chemoradiotherapy. Last, as complete response rates to neoadjuvant therapies improve, how does this affect cancer treatment? The purpose of this article is to delve into some of these matters and address them outlining the approach taken in a multidisciplinary program of rectal cancer management in a community cancer center.

The treatment of rectal cancer in 2011 has progressed dramatically. After 2 decades of discussions regarding the timing of chemotherapy and radiation, there is general consensus among rectal cancer experts that both have enormous utility in the preoperative setting.[3–9] That being stated, there is a great deal of discussion regarding the specifics of both modalities.

With regard to radiation therapy, major questions revolve around when it needs to be used, short-course versus long-course radiation,[10] and how high a dose should be given to optimize the utility of the treatment with the least morbidity to the patient.[11] In addition, newer regimens call into question how the treatment should be fractionated.

Beyond the decision of which type of chemotherapeutic agent is chosen, we need to consider the route of administration, whether given orally or intravenously, and if intravenously if given in a bolus or via continuous venous infusion. But even more generally, despite all current enthusiasm for neoadjuvant therapy we must still consider which situations arise where neoadjuvant therapy is ultimately not necessary.

Most recently, the Medical Research Council (MRC) published their results regarding routine short-course preoperative radiotherapy versus selective postoperative chemoradiotherapy for rectal cancer.[12] This study was a randomized trial including 80 centers in 4 countries with a total of 1350 patients diagnosed with operable adenocarcinoma of the rectum. What this study found was that for all stages of disease there were lower local recurrence rates at the 5-year interval using short-course preoperative radiation therapy versus selective postoperative chemoradiation. These results were quite dramatic, with a decrease from 6% to 0% local recurrence in the preoperatively treated group for stage 1 disease, 12% to 2% for stage 2 disease, and 25% to 10% for stage 3 disease when compared with patients who underwent postoperative radiotherapy (**Figs. 1** and **2**). These data argue soundly for the preoperative use of radiation therapy for all stages of disease, even patients with stage 1 rectal cancer.

As to the exact dose to be used, high-dose radiation is needed to be effective in the treatment of rectal cancer (4500 cGy). This was the dose we started using in 1976;

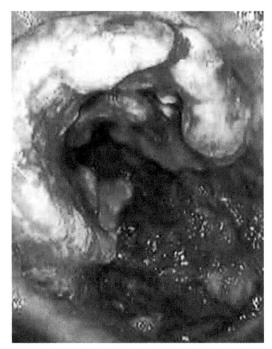

Fig. 1. Rectal cancer before neoadjuvant chemoradiation.

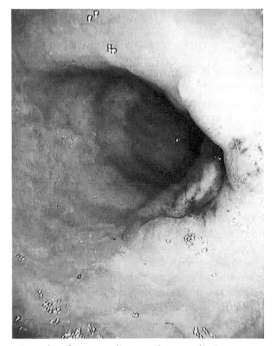

Fig. 2. Rectal cancer 6 weeks after neoadjuvant chemoradiation.

however, we now favor as a routine, the dosage of 5580 cGy. This is based on our experience published from our time at Thomas Jefferson University, where we examined our local failures and found a decreased recurrence rate with a presacral boost of treatment.[13] The intellectual basis of this has to do with the radiation sensitivity in rectal cancer and a dose response curve that shows clearly that there is a marked increase in the slope of response showing between 4500 cGy and 5500 cGy with a concomitant 50% reduction in pelvic relapse.[14]

To better communicate the tumor sensitivity in response to radiotherapy, tumor regression grading (TRG) has been added to the pathologic evaluation of rectal cancer after neoadjuvant therapy, giving a sense of the tumor's sensitivity and response to radiotherapy.[15] A TRG of 1 corresponds to minor regression of cancer, but there remains a dominant tumor mass with obvious fibrosis. A TRG of 2 corresponds to moderate regression with obvious fibrosis of the dominant tumor, with regression of 20% to 50% of the tumor. TRG 3 shows a good regression with dominant fibrosis and/or mucous substance outgrowing the tumor mass with regression of more than 50% of the tumor. TRG of 4 corresponds to a complete pathologic response.

Although this phenomenon of tumor regression has piqued the interests of many students of these studies for some time, more recently this effect has been linked to outcomes. A tumor that demonstrates a high grade of regression after neoadjuvant therapy followed by curative resection has led to improvement in overall survival. In a study by Rödel and colleagues,[16] which was a follow-up analysis of a large prospective randomized trial comparing adjuvant and neoadjuvant therapy for locally advanced rectal cancer in Germany,[5] it was shown that the patients who demonstrated a complete response to neoadjuvant radiotherapy (TRG 4) had an 86% 5-year survival rate compared with a 63% 5-year survival rate for patients with no regression or minor regression of tumor (TRG 0 and TRG 1 patients, respectively). This has focused our attention on trying to optimize tumor response to high-dose preoperative chemoradiotherapy. Although this represents an exciting field of interest, what remains to be seen is whether complete responses (CR) represent the selection of the most favorable rectal cancers or if this is altering the natural course of the disease.

The surgical management of rectal cancer is a large focus of our discussion, especially that of sphincter preservation in the distal third of the rectum. In viewing the treatment algorithm of rectal cancer from a surgical perspective, the first discussion involves whether sphincter-preservation surgery or an abdominal perineal resection with permanent end colostomy is appropriate, how to extend the performance of sphincter preservation, and what is the role of local excision. Additionally, in the age of minimally invasive surgery one must ask, what is the role of laparoscopy?

Sir Earnest Miles in 1907 reported on an abdominal perineal resection for the curative therapy of rectal cancer.[17] Although this work was a tremendous advance in the treatment of patients with rectal cancer, it unfortunately remains the dominant approach to rectal cancer for the next 100 years. Although positively affecting local recurrence rates and survival in the treatment of rectal cancer, it affected the patients' quality of life and body image at an extremely high premium. Foremost in the thoughts of the patient with low rectal cancer is avoidance of a permanent colostomy.

The challenges of rectal cancer surgery revolve around the anatomic confines of the bony pelvis. The inability to excise things laterally and the difficulty in reaching deep into the pelvis make it technically challenging to excise the cancer and perform an anastomosis, leaving the sphincter muscle intact. Although distal tumor margins are obviously a justifiable concern, the focus over recent years has rightly shifted toward obtaining clean lateral (or radial) margins as well.[18] After preoperative radiation, the challenge of excising a tumor has been compounded by the loss of a palpable mass. This can result in the inability to be confident about the tumor's location as the surgeon attempts to grasp below the cancer and adequately place a surgical clamp or stapling device.

The issue of proper margins surrounding rectal cancer has been highlighted by works published in the pathology field. In 1986, Philip Quirke and colleagues[18] published a seminal work on the subject of examining margins of patients with rectal cancer. His focus was not on the distal margin, as that could be achieved by cutting out the sphincter, but rather on the radial margin. In this group of 52 patients, they identified 26 patients who had low anterior resections and 26 patients who had abdominal perineal resection. A disappointing 30% of patients had spread to their radial margins. This was equally shared by the low anterior resection and APR groups. Of the patients who had a positive lateral margin, 75% of these patients developed a recurrence. Only one of the patients without circumferential margin positivity developed a recurrence, giving a local recurrence rate of only 3% in the negative margin group.

To understand this phenomenon better, let us look at the geometry of the entire pelvis. The bony pelvis creates a funnel filled by the cylindrical tissue of the rectum and mesorectum. As the funnel narrows, the space between the bony sidewall and the mesorectum containing the cancer becomes much smaller. With this in mind, it becomes obvious to see why it is the lateral margins rather than the distal margins where problems with adequate margins arise (**Fig. 3**).

Surgical technique matters. Although this is an inherently obvious point in the operative treatment of all visceral cancers, it has been brought to the forefront as a central issue in rectal cancer and its effective treatment. The most important day in the treatment of any patient with rectal cancer is their operative day. The need for a complete oncologic resection is paramount. A multitude of trials designed and funded nationally control very tightly radiation and chemotherapeutic parameters, but treat the operating room as a black box where no one is sure what has happened. R.J. Heald should be credited for refocusing attention on optimal operative technique and its impact on rectal surgery. In the *Journal of the Royal Society of Medicine* in 1988, he described eloquently the "Holy Plane" of Rectal Surgery.[19] This has come to be known as total mesorectal excision (TME). Although many in the United States and elsewhere in the world consider this a statement of current good oncologic rectal surgery, Heald described it clearly and drew the attention of the surgical community as to what exactly a TME entails (**Figs. 4** and **5**).

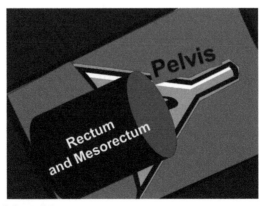

Fig. 3. Geometry of the Pelvis.

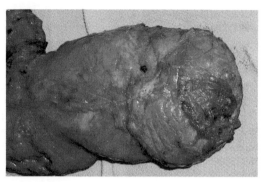

Fig. 4. Total mesorectal excision.

TOTAL MESORECTAL EXCISION

The 3 basic principles in developing this plane of dissection for a total mesorectal excision really focus on the embryologic nature of where one is working.

1. Resection of rectum and mesorectum as an intact unit using sharp dissection between the parietal and visceral planes of the pelvic fascia.
2. Visceral fascia involves the entire rectum and its mesentery.
3. Dissection in this plane reduces autonomic nerve damage and reduces local recurrence.

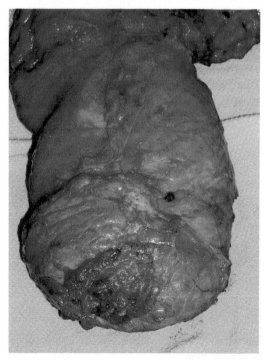

Fig. 5. Total mesorectal excision.

Resection of the rectum working in what is termed "The Holy Plane" ensures excision of the whole rectum and mesorectum as one distinct lymphovascular entity. The tumor is more apt to spread initially along the field of active lymphatic and venous flow.[20]

The cancer itself is generally limited by the embryologic envelope that the rectum itself sits in. Ultimately, as the cancer develops and progresses, if left unchecked it will grow across this and become a T4 invasive cancer. However, this is a much later stage of the disease process, and by following the 3 basic principles in developing the plane, one can usually stay out of trouble. The first principle is the recognition of mobility between the tissues of different embryologic origin. The second is the sharp dissection with good light under direct vision. The third is that of gently opening the embryologic plane with the essential addition of continuous traction on the tissues while avoiding actual tearing of the mesorectum.

Outside of the "Holy Plane" lie the autonomic nerve plexuses, pelvic veins, and internal iliac nodes. A key to the dissection is identifying the autonomic nerves and staying immediately anterior to them. There are actually 2 separate plexus planes, one inside and one outside the inferior hypogastric plexus, and by identifying the hypogastric plexus and sweeping it posteriorly, one can be reasonably sure of being directed into the proper plane (**Fig. 6**). One must then follow the nervi erigentes and pelvic plexuses and stay medial to these to avoid disturbance of sexual function while at the same time maintaining a proper oncologic resection.

Heald's contributions in the description of the technique of total mesorectal excision cannot be overstated in the treatment of rectal cancer. First, he described his own personal low local recurrence rates, roughly 50% less than what was being reported in the literature at the time.[21] But subsequently, large population studies with national audits of rectal cancer outcomes were performed showing surgeons who were trained in proper TME technique demonstrated marked diminution of their local recurrence rates. This effect was shown in the Norwegian Rectal Cancer Project, which addressed the issue of TME directly.[22] In this study, surgeons were educated about proper TME, including master classes with R.J. Heald. These surgeons reported performance rates of a proper TME as 78% in 1994 increasing to 92% in 1997. Isolated local recurrence rates were 4% for patients receiving TME versus 9% for patients without TME. In addition, this correlated with an improvement in overall survival after TME, with 5-year survival rates of 73% after TME versus 60% after conventional surgery.

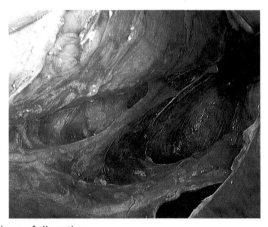

Fig. 6. Posterior plane of dissection.

The quality of oncologic resection has clearly been acted on by attention to total mesorectal excision, and the result has been an improvement in overall oncologic care. The next step forward in the treatment of patients with rectal cancer has to be improving their quality of life. Clearly nothing affects as greatly the quality of life of a patient with rectal cancer as the ability to avoid permanent colostomy and maintain normal function. The challenge in operating on a low rectal cancer during the abdominal approach is how to get beneath the cancer and perform an anastomosis. In the upper rectum, this is nonproblematic and from a technical standpoint is quite similar to a sigmoid or rectosigmoid excision. Resections that include the distal rectum are where the troubles lie from a technical standpoint for the surgeon.

Compounding this challenge is the question "what is an adequate margin for a distal rectal cancer." Every decade an additional maxim seems to be put forward and one debunked. Originally there was a 5-cm rule postulated as necessary for proper oncologic resection.[23] This was then revised to a 2-cm rule in the 1990s.[24] In the early portion of this century the question that has been raised is whether less than a 1-cm margin is sufficient so long as it is an R0 resection.[25–28] The reason that this discussion is germane relates to the persistently high incidence of abdominal perineal resection. The original Swedish rectal cancer trial published in the *New England Journal of Medicine* in 1997 involved 908 patients treated with surgery alone versus surgery and radiation. Both cohorts had an APR rate of more than 50%.[3] The last major rectal cancer management trial published in the United States (NSABP R-03 Trial) had to be halted because of lack of accrual. However, in the preoperative radiotherapy group, APR rates were 50% and even higher in the surgery-alone arm.[29] The German Rectal Cancer Trial (CRO-CAO-A10-94) showed an APR rate of 61% in the preoperative radiotherapy group compared with an APR rate of 81% in the postoperative radiotherapy group ($P = .004$).[30] In the Polish colorectal study group, APR rates were 40% in both the short- and long-course radiotherapy group.[10] With data such as these as a background, it is understandable why there is such concern in the medical and lay communities regarding the need for a permanent colostomy in the care of patients with rectal cancer.

Against this background, we consider our program of rectal cancer in a teaching, community hospital center. Our rectal cancer management program using high-dose radiotherapy originates in 1976 at Thomas Jefferson University. This represents the first experience of sphincter-preserving surgery after high-dose preoperative irradiation.[31] It is worth noting that at the time many considered it malpractice to even operate on the pelvis after irradiation, because of concerns in the 1970s regarding morbidity and mortality when operating in the irradiated field.

There are 6 keys to extending sphincter preservation in rectal cancer management. This approach, originally developed at Jefferson, and currently used in a community colorectal surgical unit at our hospital, includes 6 factors that must be incorporated to alter the rate of sphincter preservation (**Fig. 7**). If our goal is to decrease APR rates from 40% to 60%, as noted in the major national trials discussed earlier, to 7% in our experience, we need to focus on the following:

1. Using higher radiation therapy doses, on average now to 5580 cGy.
   As explained earlier, this relatively small escalation in radiation dose has an exaggerated effect on tumor regression, which we are able to take advantage of.[13]
2. Base decisions on sphincter preservation on the status of the cancer AFTER completion of chemoradiotherapy.

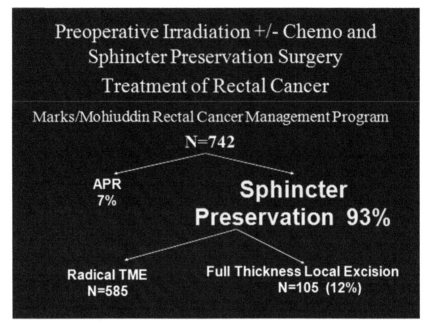

Fig. 7. Rectal cancer management program.

Although this is a basic tenet of our rectal cancer management program at Lankenau Hospital, it represents a major departure for many. The oncologic community (surgical and medical) has been taught that it is the initial presentation of the cancer that will dictate subsequent treatment. This lack of plasticity of thought has hindered surgeons from reaping perhaps the most significant benefit of tumor downstaging for rectal cancer after chemoradiation, the preservation of the sphincter. Let us be clear that the dictum that treatment must be based on the initial presentation of the cancer where sphincter preservation hangs in the balance for many low rectal cancers, must be abandoned. Downstaging after neoadjuvant therapy clearly has a dramatic effect on surgical options.

3. Accepting distal margins of resection from the cancer as small as 5 mm in length. Although we are certainly not advocates for minimal margins for cancers in the proximal rectum, for adenocarcinomas of the distal 3 cm of the rectum accepting smaller distal margins on an otherwise R0 resection allows us to apply sphincter-preservation techniques in situations that would not be possible if the 2-cm rule was invoked. This strategy, as you will see, has been supported with impressive oncologic results.

4. Extended interval between completion of radiation therapy and surgery (8–12 weeks). Although we are in the process of researching this point, it has been our strong clinical impression that by extending this period from our original 6- to 8-week period following radiation to 8 to 12 weeks, additional downstaging occurs. With this further tumor regression comes improved applicability of sphincter preservation.

5. Transanal abdominal transanal proctosigmoidectomy (TATA) surgical technique. This operation allows for the creation of a known distal margin to the cancer even after downstaging. This technique, only for cancers of the distal 3 cm of the rectum, combats both the difficulty of obtaining a safe margin as well as the ability to perform a low anastomosis.

6. Full-thickness local excision (FTLE).

This is another technique that allows for distal rectal cancers to be excised with sphincter preservation, also taking advantage of the downstaging that occurs after chemoirradiation. FTLE is used only for select tumors that have an excellent response to chemoradiation therapy.

Our treatment algorithm is shown in **Fig. 8**. This is the selection scheme that we use for all patients with rectal cancer. First, all patients are examined digitally and with flexible and/or rigid endoscopy. The level of the tumor is assessed and recorded relative to the anorectal ring, which is the terminal aspect of the rectum and the superior border of the anal canal. In addition, we assess the level from the anal verge; however, this is a highly variable data point because the length of the anal canal can vary substantially depending on the body habitus and weight of the patient. With digital examination as well as the addition of office flexible and at times rigid sigmoidoscopy, we assess the size of the tumor, the clinical T stage, depth, the presence and depth of ulceration, mobility or fixity of the cancer, the shape of the lesion, and its position in the rectum. These characteristics are all prospectively recorded. Patients routinely undergo endoscopic ultrasound, MRI of the pelvis, or both for further staging. MRI is routinely used in cancers with obstructing components.

Radiation therapy is used for all cancers in the distal 6 cm of the rectum as well as unfavorable cancers. An unfavorable cancer is defined as stage T3 or a cancer that demonstrates node positivity. Although modified depending on individual patient factors, the standard treatment is to 5580 cGy. This includes 4500 cGY treatment to the pelvis with an additional boost to the presacral region and/or the area of the tumor.[13] Chemotherapy is 5FU based and although it can be bolus or oral in form, is generally continues venous infusion.

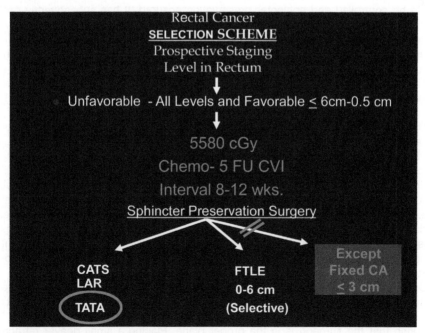

Fig. 8. Treatment selection algorithm.

After neoadjuvant therapy is complete, there is an interval of 8 to 12 weeks before making a final decision regarding sphincter preservation. We see the patient in 3-week intervals during and following therapy to ensure that there is proper tumor response and whether an additional boost to the tumor may be necessary. Any subsequent therapy also depends on how the patient is tolerating the treatment.

Between 8 and 12 weeks after completion of radiotherapy, the patient undergoes another complete examination including digital rectal examination and flexible endoscopic evaluation to reassess all the parameters that have been originally noted, and picture of the tumor after radiotherapy. It is at this point that we make a final decision regarding the applicability of sphincter preservation. All cancers except those that remain fixed in the distal 3 cm of the rectum undergo sphincter-preservation surgery. For those cancers that remain fixed in the distal 3 cm, abdominal perineal resection is performed. Sphincter-preservation surgery is performed via radical resection with temporary diverting colostomy or ileostomy, or a full-thickness local excision with transanal endoscopic microsurgery (TEM).

SPHINCTER-PRESERVATION SURGERY
TATA

The TATA (transanal abdominal transanal proctosigmoidectomy descending coloanal anastomosis and diverting loop stoma) is an original operation first developed and performed by Dr Gerald Marks in 1984. At that time, it was noted that in the very low rectum it was difficult to palpate the location of the cancer after the cancer had been downstaged from high-dose preoperative radiotherapy.[32] This led Dr Gerald Marks to the cadaver lab where he developed a technique to address this problem. He titled this a transanal abdominal transanal proctosigmoidectomy with descending coloanal anastomosis or TATA.[33] The unique technical aspect of this operation was that the operation was started transanally so there was a known distal margin that could be controlled and sphincter preservation ensured. It has subsequently been referred to in publications from other centers as an intersphincteric proctectomy. As stated previously, the ability to obtain a known distal margin at the beginning of the operation transanally facilitates a precise distal dissection of the cancer. This assuages both the challenge of an impalpable scar after chemoradiation as well as the issue of trying to successfully place a clamp distal to it. Additionally, this approach allows us to state with confidence preoperatively if sphincter preservation will be accomplishable, facilitating a well-informed conversation with the patient.

The procedure commences with the patient in extended lithotomy position. Before initiation of the dissection of the rectum, povidone-iodine (Betadine) or even a dilute povidone-iodine (Betadine)-soaked sponge can be placed into the anal canal. Once this is done, we avoid placing a finger in the rectum to minimize the possibility of implanting tumor cells. Next, Alice-Adair clamps are placed circumferentially around the anal canal to evert the anal tissue and allow visualization of the dentate line. Electrocautery is used to incise at the dentate line through the mucosa circumferentially. This avoids a vertical linear tear to the rectal wall during the full thickness dissection. The dissection continues perpendicular to the rectal wall to enter into the plane between the full thickness of the rectum, which at this level really is the upper portion of the internal sphincter, down to the puborectalis.

Once this plane is developed, the Alice-Adair clamps are applied to the transected distal portion of the rectum, and using the scissors, the shiny glistening white aspect of the puborectalis can be identified. Visualization of this white tissue is the key to ensuring that the surgeon is in the proper plane. Placing a small deaver retractor allows development of the plane between the rectum and the Levator-ani complex. The dissection is brought around anteriorly in sharp fashion. In women, a finger in the vagina allows appreciation of the vaginal wall, and avoidance of this structure is generally not a problem. In male patients, one has to be careful as the dissection is taken anteriorly, to avoid proceeding anterior to the prostate. However, paying close attention to the region between the prostate and the rectum clarifies the space between them and this space opens readily. The length of dissection cephalad is taken up to the seminal vesicles generally in the male patient and the cervix in the female patient. Once this is completed, the rectum itself is oversewn in an airtight fashion with an 0-vicryl stitch turning the edges inward so as to avoid fecal spillage or potential spillage of cancer cells during the abdominal phase of the operation. Following completion of this, the pelvis is irrigated from below and a lap pad or e-tape is placed through the anus.

The operation then begins abdominally. This is performed in either an open or laparoscopic fashion. In both procedures, a total mesorectal excision is performed. Key components of the abdominal operation include the following:

1. Full release of the splenic flexure, with dissection of the transverse colon mesentery off the inferior border of the pancreas to allow optimal mobility of the colon for a low anastomosis.
2. Resection of the entirety of the rectum and sigmoid colon up to the distal-most descending colon. This ensures that any irradiated colon has been removed with the specimen. The sigmoid colon often falls down into the pelvis and can be expected to receive some radiation even though attempts are made to exclude it from the field. As such, we always mark the junction of the descending colon and sigmoid colon with a stitch before any mobilization, which may obscure this landmark.
3. High ligation of the inferior mesenteric artery (IMA) after identification of the left ureter. This portion of the operation is facilitated by identifying the hypogastric nerves and sweeping them posteriorly, which places one in the proper plane to identify both the ureter and come around the IMA.
4. Transecting the inferior mesenteric vein (IMV) proximally and distally. It is essential that the IMV is taken and secured properly immediately inferior to the inferior border of the pancreas. This is necessary to allow for a tension-free anastomosis in the low pelvis. Attempts to preserve this venous drainage will clearly result in ischemia to the neorectum. If additional length is necessary, the mesentery is divided deeply to allow for preservation of the marginal artery.
5. Mobilization of the colon from its lateral attachments.
6. Total mesorectal excision facilitated by the prior transanal dissection. As one opens the peritoneum sharply along the length of the perirectal sulcus and anteriorly in the pouch of Douglas, the hypogastric nerves are followed and swept posteriorly. The dissection is maintained in the areolar plane immediately anterior to this. This allows protection of the embryologic envelope of the mesorectum and is the hallmark of the total mesorectal excision. This is done under direct vision with a good light and sharp dissection in this plane. Dissection is generally started posteriorly and oftentimes one can connect to the dissection from the perineum posteriorly. This facilitates bringing the dissection laterally to the right and left respecting the nervi erigentes and then easily transecting the remnant tissue anteriorly.

    This strategy is modified depending on the site of the tumor as well as its size and bulk. Bulky tumors with any adherence are addressed last after the rest of the rectum is mobilized. It is essential that this is mobilized sharply. However, when applying retraction, care must be taken not to apply too much pressure as this may tear the tumor off the adjacent sidewall. This will cause tumor fragmentation and likely result in an R1 resection.

7. If the tumor is adherent to a nonvital structure, it is resected en bloc. If the tumor is adjacent to the pelvic sidewall above the 3-cm level, this is addressed with sharp dissection, trusting in the radiotherapy to sterilize the margins. Bony prominences are left in place, assuming there is no indication of actual extension of the cancer into the periosteum itself on preoperative imaging. This uses some of the maxims described earlier of our sphincter- preservation program, which relies on assessment of the tumor after completion of radiotherapy and taking maximal benefit of downstaging.[34] The radiation effect is greatest in the periphery of the cancer, which has the highest density of vascularity and therefore the highest response to the ionizing effect of radiation.[34]

After completion of the circumferential resection of the rectum, the specimen is delivered abdominally or transanally and either a direct or colonic J-pouch coloanal hand-sewn anastomosis is performed. This is done by taking full-thickness bites through the descending colonic wall and the through the transected lower border of the internal sphincter and overlying anoderm. Four corner sutures are placed at 12, 6, 3, and 9 o'clock positions and 1 or 2 full-thickness bites are taken between these. The Cardinal sutures are left untied so that the colonic wall can be manipulated back and forth to allow good application of the suture needle. Additional sutures are placed between these to make sure that there are no gaps in the suture line. These stitches are then tied. Digital examination is performed to ensure there are no gaps and the anastomosis is patent.

Role of Laparoscopic Surgery

Into the mix of questions surrounding the proper treatment of rectal cancer is whether or not laparoscopic TME is an acceptable approach. Although careful surgical technique as discussed earlier has clearly been related to better outcomes in rectal cancer surgery, there are concerns as to whether or not laparoscopy will negatively impact this. Some controversy surrounding laparoscopic proctectomy has to do with whether the splenic flexure can be properly released and if a safe high ligation of the IMA can be performed. But most importantly, there is concern as to whether or not it is feasible to do a true total mesorectal excision laparoscopically.

In the mid to late 1990s, many leaders in the field of minimally invasive surgery and laparoscopic surgery expressed significant questions. No less an authority than R.J. Heald wrote the following with O'Rourke in the *British Journal of Surgery* in 1993, "Uncertain efficacy of laparoscopic technique and technology....believe rectal cancer....should only be operated upon by specialist colorectal surgeons in a conventional or open fashion...."[21] Köckerling and Scheidbach[35] published an editorial in 2000 stating "the rectum is not suitable generally for laparoscopic resection." These statements reflect not only a consensus view at the time but an intelligent assessment of the challenges. The fundamental challenges of laparoscopic low pelvic surgery echo those of low rectal cancer surgery in an open fashion. This has to do with the confines of the bony pelvis, the ability to obtain safe lateral, circumferential, and distal margins, as well as the technical aspects of obtaining adequate retraction and distal transection. That said, it has become clear to those of us with experience in the field that visualization is clearly improved in the deep pelvis with the addition of laparoscopy and one is able to see where one is working much more clearly with a laparoscope than in an open fashion.

Questions surrounding the application of laparoscopic techniques for cancer of both the colon and the rectum have existed from the start. Significantly, the COST trial, a comparative evaluation of laparoscopic-assisted versus open surgery for colon cancer, was published in the *New England Journal of Medicine* in May 2004.[36] This prospective, multi-institutional trial fundamentally shifted the landscape of the treatment for colon cancer overnight. By showing unequivocally that there was no negative impact in local recurrence or survival for any stage patient operated on laparoscopically, it shifted the discussion regarding the role of laparoscopy in colon surgery fundamentally. It also quelled the fears that some had about wound implantation of tumor cells, showing that there was no higher incidence in the laparoscopically treated patients. In addition, this study showed a clear benefit of quality of life in the perioperative period, a 50% decrease in the need for parenteral narcotics, and twice the need for oral narcotics as an outpatient in the open group.

With this information, many of the theoretical issues of laparoscopy had been firmly addressed. Additionally, Lawrence Whelan, MD's group at Columbia University had established that tumors grow larger and are more easily established after laparotomy rather than laparoscopy in the mouse model.[37] By opening the notion that there is a diminished immunologic suppression by less of a stress response around laparoscopic compared with open surgery, theoretically laparoscopy represents an actual advantage in the colorectal patient.

Although many of the challenges of rectal resection are common to both laparoscopic and open methods, there are specific issues unique to laparoscopic rectal surgery. These include the following:

1. How to apply the stapler in the low pelvis?
2. How to obtain adequate retraction in the pelvis for visualization?
3. How to operate in a tight space where small amounts of blood may impede adequate visualization?

To address the technical issues surrounding how to perform a laparoscopic total mesorectal excision in the low pelvis, we developed a concept of 3-dimensional retraction. The essential notion here is to recreate the directions of retraction that are obtained in an open pelvic dissection. This involves the placement of a grasper from a left lower quadrant port site to recreate the St Mark's retractor as well as a 5-mm port placed suprapubically to give lateral retraction to the right and left pelvic sidewall. We frequently use a suction device for the lateral retraction, creating tension between the embryologic planes of the mesorectum and the sidewall (**Fig. 9**).

The abdominal operation is performed in a 3-trochar technique as originally described by Huscher and Marescaux.[38] Once the abdominal portion is completed, our standardized approach for total mesorectal excision in a laparoscopic fashion centers around an organized plan:

1. Open the box of the pelvis circumferentially.
2. Dissection is taken posteriorly first.
3. This is brought around the right lateral and then the left lateral side.
4. Then it is finished anteriorly. This follows the tenets of total mesorectal excision.

To open the box, endoshears with electrocautery attached are used extending the divisional attachments along the left pelvic sidewall and the line of Toldt down along the rectal sulcus. Hook cautery is also occasionally used. This is felt to be preferential to Ligasure or Harmonic Scalpel, as it is much finer at only a millimeter in width, and precision in this area is quite important. Once the peritoneum is open on the right

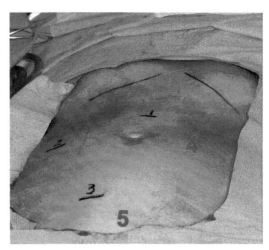

Fig. 9. Laparoscopic port placement.

side, it is then opened along the left side. The suction device is an excellent retractor coming in from the suprapubic port to create lateral retraction along the sidewall. This allows the mesorectum to stand in sharp contrast to the area of transection. The peritoneal opening is connected anteriorly with aid of the left lower quadrant port retractor, often just a fenestrated grasper, which lifts up the anterior leaf of the pouch of Douglas.

Once this is completed, the next step is to take the dissection posteriorly. To do this, the operating surgeon grasps the rectum and holds it anteriorly. The hypogastric nerves are swept posteriorly and the suction device, through the suprapubic port, is used to gain anterior and lateral retraction on the mesorectum. The suction device is activated every time the electrocautery is used. This keeps the area smoke free and diminishes the amount of blood in the field. Any amount of blood in this tight space will compound the difficulty of the dissection.

To definitively address questions regarding laparoscopic TME, the American College of Surgeons Oncology Group (ACOSOG)-Z6051 trial has been initiated. This multi-institutional prospective trial based on the Clinical Outcomes of Surgical Therapy Study Group trial organization, is under way to address the success of laparoscopic TME. To do so, 480 patients, 240 in each arm, will be operated on in a laparoscopic or open/laparoscopy-assisted fashion, where the TME is performed through an open incision but everything else can be done laparoscopically. Primary end points will be pathologic in this case:

1. Circumferential margins greater than 1 mm
2. Distal margin greater than 2 cm, greater than 1 cm distal rectum
3. Complete TME excision.

We recently reported on our laparoscopic TATA experience with the aim of looking at short-term and long-term results.[39] After exclusionary criteria, we identified 79 consecutive patients with rectal cancer who were treated with laparoscopic TATA from 1998 to 2008. All patients were diagnosed with rectal cancers within 3 cm of the anorectal ring. All patients received neoadjuvant chemoradiation. Of the 66 patients who were evaluated before neoadjuvant therapy, 50 patients were staged as T3 and 16 patients were staged as T2. The remaining 13 patients had already completed their neoadjuvant therapy before presentation at our clinic. The mean level in the rectum for all patients was 1.2 cm. Thirty-one tumors were mobile, 27 were tethered, and 8 showed early fixation. The mean external beam radiation dose was 5400 cGy and 77 patients underwent concurrent chemotherapy.

The mean follow-up period was 34 months. There were no mortalities. The overall laparoscopic completion rate was 94.9%. After surgery, pathologic review of the specimens revealed 22 complete responses (28%), 12 ypT1 cancers (15%), 22 ypT2 cancers (29%), and 23 ypT3 cancers (29%). Fourteen cancers were node-positive (17%). One patient had a positive distal margin (1.3%). Six patients had positive circumferential margins (6.3%).

Local recurrence rate was 2.5% (2/79) and the distant metastasis rate was 10.1% (8/79). Overall, 90% of patients lived without a stoma. Causes for neorectal loss were ischemia of the neorectum (2 patients, 2.5%), local recurrence, or positive margins (3 patients, 3.7%). Two patients did not have their condition reversed owing to comorbidities and one patient had a stoma secondary to bowel obstruction.

The overall Kaplan-Meier 5-year actuarial survival rate was 97%, which compares favorably with the literature. Multiple studies have shown local recurrence rates from 4% to 17% after chemoradiation for low rectal cancers.[11,40–43] Even though these studies typically involve higher lesions that carry a better prognosis and lower risk of local recurrence, our results compare favorably. These long-term data support the oncologic basis for the intersphincteric dissection performed during the TATA procedure. A local recurrence rate of only 2.5%, although accomplishing sphincter preservation for cancer in the distal 3 cm of the rectum, reinforces the need to base decisions on the postirradiated rectal cancer to allow extension of sphincter preservation.

Local Excision

The ultimate in minimally invasive treatment of rectal cancer is really that of full-thickness local excision. In 1984, our unit was the first to perform and report on a full-thickness local excision of rectal cancer after irradiation therapy.[44] The first case was in a medically frail patient who would not stand radical surgery. The questions at the time were whether the wound would heal, what function the patient would maintain, and what cancer control would be provided.

In 2003, we reported on our experience with 83 patients after preoperative radiation and chemotherapy. Selection criteria for this group were based again on the reassessment of the cancer after completion of radiation therapy. For patients whose cancer was judged to be confined to the rectal wall without nodal involvement, a local excision was offered. The treatment categories consisted of 2 groups: (1) medically compromised and (2) elective or staged category. The group of patients who were medically compromised would not undergo any additional surgery, even if their pathology revealed more-advanced cancer. The second group, the elective or staged category of patients who either because of their refusal for radical surgery or their comorbid diseases, a local excision was considered optimal. In this group of patients, the FTLE effectively represented an excisional biopsy. If a full-thickness cancer (ie, ypT3 cancer) or node-positive cancer was found, these patients were referred for radical surgery. Often patients in the staged group had a challenging body habitus or extensive diverticular disease that made them not prohibitive candidates for radical surgery but certainly candidates who would benefit significantly from less invasive therapies with less risk of significant morbidities. It is worth noting that in this original group of 83 patients, 2 of 3 had been recommended for an APR before being seen by us and 63% had their tumors located in the distal 3 cm of the rectum.

The operations performed were transanal, transphincteric, transacral, and since 1998 transanal endoscopic microsurgery has been used. In this patient population, 88% of the patients were able to have their cancer definitively treated without the need for a stoma. Two patients had advanced cancers and went on to APRs. One patient, a thin diabetic woman, with an anterior-based cancer developed a recto-vaginal fistula. One patient had a stoma because of incontinence, and 4 patients had diversion because of recurrent disease (2 for APR and 2 were just diverted). Overall, in this treatment group there was a 12% recurrence rate and an impressive 4% for the TEM group.

SUMMARY

In summary, advances in neoadjuvant therapy in the treatment of rectal cancer promises to further expand curative options for patients with rectal cancer without the need for a permanent colostomy. Local excision, especially using TEM surgery, has the potential to be widely applicable. Challenges exist in the prospective evaluation regarding nodal involvement. Additional work is going to be required for identifying patients with node-negative versus node-positive disease with a focus on salvage rates and ultimate stoma rates with this approach.

Minimally invasive surgery will clearly play a role in rectal cancer management in the hands of experienced laparoscopic rectal cancer surgeons. This is something that the ACOSOG-Z6501 trial should demonstrate definitively. Last, and most important, sphincter- preservation surgery can be extended in the distal third of the rectum with attention and individualization of care using advances in radiation, chemotherapy, and surgical techniques. As we have done, this can certainly be achieved within the confines of a community center with a dedicated focus on rectal cancer. Although specialist care is often associated in the minds of the public with a university, it is well to remember that patients are cared for by individuals and individuals can work in university or community settings. With a dedicated team and a multidisciplinary approach, expert care can be given to patients with cancer even in the most distal rectum while maintaining their quality of life, avoiding a permanent colostomy, and providing excellent rates of local control and survival.

REFERENCES

1. Altekruse S, Kosary C, Krapcho M, et al. SEER Cancer statistics review 1975–2007. Bethesda (MD): National Cancer Institute; 2009.
2. The American Cancer Society Society AC. What are the key statistics about colorectal cancer? in 2010, vol. 2010. Available at: http://www.cancer.org/cancer/colonandrectumcancer/detailedguide/colorectal-cancer-key-statistics. Accessed January 25, 2011.
3. Payhlman L, Glimelius B. Improved survival with preoperative radiotherapy in resectable rectal cancer. Swedish Rectal Cancer Trial. N Engl J Med 1997;336: 980.
4. Crane C, Skibber J, Birnbaum E, et al. The addition of continuous infusion 5-FU to preoperative radiation therapy increases tumor response, leading to increased sphincter preservation in locally advanced rectal cancer. Int J Radiat Oncol Biol Phys 2003;57:84.
5. Sauer R, Becker H, Hohenberger W, et al. Preoperative versus postoperative chemoradiotherapy for rectal cancer. N Engl J Med 2004;351:1731.
6. Randomized study on preoperative radiotherapy in rectal carcinoma. Stockholm Colorectal Cancer Study Group. Ann Surg Oncol 1996;3:423.
7. Roh M, Colangelo L, Wieand S, et al. Response to preoperative multimodality therapy predicts survival in patients with carcinoma of the rectum. J Clin Oncol 2004;22:3505.

8. Bosset J, Collette L, Calais G, et al. Chemotherapy with preoperative radiotherapy in rectal cancer. N Engl J Med 2006;355:1114.

9. Gérard J, Conroy T, Bonnetain F, et al. Preoperative radiotherapy with or without concurrent fluorouracil and leucovorin in T3-4 rectal cancers: results of FFCD 9203. J Clin Oncol 2006;24:4620.

10. Chmielik E, Bujko K, Nasierowska-Guttmejer A, et al. Distal intramural spread of rectal cancer after preoperative radiotherapy: the results of a multicenter randomized clinical study. Int J Radiat Oncol Biol Phys 2006;65:182.

11. Mohiuddin M, Regine W, Marks G, et al. High-dose preoperative radiation and the challenge of sphincter-preservation surgery for cancer of the distal 2 cm of the rectum. Int J Radiat Oncol Biol Phys 1998;40:569.

12. Sebag-Montefiore D, Quirke P, Steele R, et al. The impact of short course preoperative radiotherapy on patients' quality of life: data from the MRC CR07/ NCIC CO16 randomised clinical trial in patients with rectal cancer. Int J Radiat Oncol Biol Phys 2008;72:S28.

13. Mohiuddin M, Marks G. Patterns of recurrence following high-dose preoperative radiation and sphincter-preserving surgery for cancer of the rectum. Dis Colon Rectum 1993;36:117.

14. Suwinski R, Taylor J, Withers H. Rapid growth of microscopic rectal cancer as a determinant of response to preoperative radiation therapy. Int J Radiat Oncol Biol Phys 1998;42:943.

15. Dworak O, Keilholz L, Hoffmann A. Pathological features of rectal cancer after preoperative radiochemotherapy. Int J Colorectal Dis 1997;12:19.

16. Rödel C, Martus P, Papadoupolos T, et al. Prognostic significance of tumor regression after preoperative chemoradiotherapy for rectal cancer. J Clin Oncol 2005;23:8688.

17. Miles W. A method of performing abdomino-perineal excision for carcinoma of the rectum and of the terminal portion of the pelvic colon. Lancet 1812;2:1908.

18. Quirke P, Durdey P, Dixon M, et al. Local recurrence of rectal adenocarcinoma due to inadequate surgical resection. Histopathological study of lateral tumour spread and surgical excision. Lancet 1986;2:996.

19. Heald R. The "Holy Plane" of rectal surgery. J R Soc Med 1988;81:503.

20. Zheng Y, Zhou Z, Li L, et al. Distribution and patterns of lymph node metastases and micrometastases in the mesorectum of rectal cancer. J Surg Oncol 2007;96:213.

21. O'Rourke N, Heald R. Laparoscopic surgery for colorectal cancer. Br J Surg 1993;80:1229.

22. Wibe A, Møller B, Norstein J, et al. A national strategic change in treatment policy for rectal cancer—implementation of total mesorectal excision as routine treatment in Norway. A national audit. Dis Colon Rectum 2002;45:857.

23. Feil W, Wunderlich M, Kovats E, et al. Rectal cancer: factors influencing the development of local recurrence after radical anterior resection. Int J Colorectal Dis 1988;3:195.

24. Williams NS, Dixon MF, Johnston D. Reappraisal of the 5 centimetre rule of distal excision for carcinoma of the rectum: a study of distal intramural spread and of patients' survival. Br J Surg 1983;70:150.

25. Moore H, Riedel E, Minsky B, et al. Adequacy of 1-cm distal margin after restorative rectal cancer resection with sharp mesorectal excision and preoperative combined-modality therapy. Ann Surg Oncol 2003;10:80.

26. Kuvshinoff B, Maghfoor I, Miedema B, et al. Distal margin requirements after preoperative chemoradiotherapy for distal rectal carcinomas: are < or = 1 cm distal margins sufficient? Ann Surg Oncol 2001;8:163.

27. Karanjia ND, Schache DJ, North WR, et al. "Close shave" in anterior resection. Br J Surg 1990;77:510.

28. Shirouzu K, Isomoto H, Kakegawa T. Distal spread of rectal cancer and optimal distal margin of resection for sphincter-preserving surgery. Cancer 1995;76:388.

29. Hyams D, Mamounas E, Petrelli N, et al. A clinical trial to evaluate the worth of preoperative multimodality therapy in patients with operable carcinoma of the rectum: a progress report of National Surgical Breast and Bowel Project Protocol R-03. Dis Colon Rectum 1997;40:131.

30. Sauer R, Fietkau R, Wittekind C, et al. Adjuvant vs. neoadjuvant radiochemotherapy for locally advanced rectal cancer: the German trial CAO/ARO/AIO-94. Colorectal Dis 2003;5:406.

31. Marks G, Mohiuddin M, Borenstein B. Preoperative radiation therapy and sphincter preservation by the combined abdominotranssacral technique for selected rectal cancers. Dis Colon Rectum 1985;28:565.

32. Marks G. Combined abdominotranssacral reconstruction of the radiation-injured rectum. Am J Surg 1976;131:54.

33. Marks G, Bannon J, Marks J. Transanal-abdominal transanal-radical proctosigmoidectomy with coloanal anastomosis for distal rectal cancer. In: Baker R, Fischer J, Nyhus L, editors. Mastery of surgery. 3rd edition. Boston (MA): Little, Brown and Company Inc; 1996. p. 1524–34.

34. Konerding M, Fait E, Gaumann A. 3D microvascular architecture of precancerous lesions and invasive carcinomas of the colon. Br J Surg 2001;84:1354.

35. Köckerling F, Scheidbach H. Current status of laparoscopic surgery. Surg Endosc 2000;14:777.

36. Nelson H, Sargent D, Wieand H. A comparison of laparoscopically assisted and open colectomy for colon cancer. N Engl J Med 2004;350:2050.

37. Allendorf J, Bessler M, Horvath K, et al. Increased tumor establishment and growth after open vs laparoscopic bowel resection in mice. Surg Endosc 1998;12:1035.

38. Huscher C, Marescaux J. Three port technique for laparoscopic left colectomy. WeBSurg; 2009. Available at: http://www.websurg.com/ref/media.php?doi=vd01en2635&nohead=1. Accessed January 25, 2011.

39. Marks J, Mizrahi B, Dalane S, et al. Laparoscopic transanal abdominal transanal resection with sphincter preservation for rectal cancer in the distal 3 cm of the rectum after neoadjuvant therapy. Surg Endosc 2010;24(11):2700–7.

40. Rullier E, Goffre B, Bonnel C, et al. Preoperative radiochemotherapy and sphincter-saving resection for T3 carcinomas of the lower third of the rectum. Ann Surg 2001;234:633.

41. Marks G, Mohiuddin M, Masoni L. The reality of radical sphincter preservation surgery for cancer of the distal 3 cm of rectum following high-dose radiation. Int J Radiat Oncol Biol Phys 1993;27:779.

42. Rouanet P, Fabre J, Dubois J, et al. Conservative surgery for low rectal carcinoma after high-dose radiation: functional and oncologic results. Ann Surg 1995;221:67.

43. Wagman R, Minsky B, Cohen A, et al. Sphincter preservation in rectal cancer with preoperative radiation therapy and coloanal anastomosis: long term follow-up. Int J Radiat Oncol Biol Phys 1998;42:51.

44. Marks G, Mohiuddin M, Masoni L, et al. High-dose preoperative radiation and full-thickness local excision. A new option for patients with select cancers of the rectum. Dis Colon Rectum 1990;33:735.

Minimally Invasive Esophagectomy in the Community Hospital Setting

Erin M. Hanna, MD[a], H. James Norton, PhD[b],
Mark K. Reames, MD[c], Jonathan C. Salo, MD[d],*

KEYWORDS

• Esophagectomy • Minimally invasive • Esophageal cancer
• Community hospital

Although associated with substantial morbidity and mortality, esophagectomy remains the preferred treatment for resectable esophageal cancer. Minimally invasive techniques have been used for esophagectomy in an effort to reduce the morbidity and mortality of this complex operation. In this report, the authors describe their experience with minimally invasive esophagectomy (MIE) at Carolinas Medical Center, a community academic medical center serving western North Carolina and northern South Carolina.

MIE describes the use of laparoscopic or thoracoscopic techniques to mobilize the esophagus for resection and restoration of gastrointestinal continuity. These techniques were derived after recognizing the significant postoperative morbidity and mortality associated with traditional open esophageal resection. Rates of postoperative morbidity from the traditional open esophageal resection range as high as 40% to 60% with mortality rates of 5% to 20%.[1] With the likelihood of postoperative complications, surgeons have sought to find new and different approaches with the goal of lowering overall morbidity and mortality.

OPEN ESOPHAGECTOMY TECHNIQUES

The 3 most commonly performed open esophagectomy procedures are the transhiatal esophagectomy, transthoracic (Ivor Lewis) esophagectomy, and the 3-stage

Statement of Disclosure: The authors have nothing to disclose.
[a] Department of General Surgery, Carolinas Medical Center, 1000 Blythe Boulevard, PO Box 32861, Charlotte, NC 28232-2861, USA
[b] Department of Biostatistics, Carolinas Medical Center, 1000 Blythe Boulevard, PO Box 32861, Charlotte, NC 28232-2861, USA
[c] Sanger Heart and Vascular Institute, 1000 Blythe Boulevard Suite 300, Charlotte, NC 28203, USA
[d] Division of Surgical Oncology, Department of General Surgery, Carolinas Medical Center – Blumenthal Cancer Center, 1025 Morehead Medical Drive, Charlotte, NC 28204, USA
* Corresponding author.
E-mail address: Jonathan.salo@carolinashealthcare.org

Surg Oncol Clin N Am 20 (2011) 521–530
doi:10.1016/j.soc.2011.01.009
1055-3207/11/$ – see front matter © 2011 Published by Elsevier Inc.

surgonc.theclinics.com

(McKeown) esophagectomy. All 3 operations begin with a midline laparotomy for mobilization of the stomach and formation of a gastric conduit. A transhiatal esophagectomy uses a cervical incision to mobilize the cervical esophagus. The thoracic esophagus is then mobilized by blunt dissection from the abdominal and cervical incisions. The gastric conduit is brought up to the neck and a cervical anastomosis constructed. Transthoracic esophagectomy uses a right thoracotomy to mobilize and remove the esophagus and allow creation of an intrathoracic anastomosis. A 3-stage esophagectomy uses a right thoracotomy for mobilization of the esophagus, but in addition removes the proximal esophagus and creates a cervical anastomosis.

MINIMALLY INVASIVE ESOPHAGECTOMY TECHNIQUES

Increasing experience with laparoscopic surgery in the 1990s led to the development of MIE techniques. The precursor to this was the thoracoscopic mobilization of the esophagus in 1992 by Cuschieri and colleagues.[2] Later work by Dallemagne[3] combined laparoscopic and thoracoscopic resection of esophageal cancer, which led to the current techniques used in MIE. In modern practice, the 3 most frequently performed procedures for MIE include the thoracoscopic/laparoscopic esophagectomy with a cervical anastomosis, thoracoscopic/laparoscopic Ivor Lewis esophagectomy, and laparoscopic transhiatal esophagectomy with a cervical anastomosis. Many variations in technique have been described.

MINIMALLY INVASIVE VERSUS OPEN ESOPHAGECTOMY

To date, no randomized trials have compared outcomes of esophageal resection using a minimally invasive approach with open esophagectomy.[4] Several nonrandomized comparative reports have been published, which have generally compared the two techniques with the same institution, often using historical experience within open esophagectomy. A meta-analysis of 12 comparative reports encompassing 672 MIEs and 612 open esophagectomies found shorter hospital stay, less blood loss, and fewer complications with MIE.[5] An analysis of 1008 patients in 8 comparative studies[6] found equivalent outcomes with the exceptions of higher stricture rate among MIE and lower overall morbidity after MIE compared with open esophagectomy. A retrospective review of 699 MIEs conducted in England between 1996 and 2008 found lower in-hospital, 30-day, and 365-day mortality as compared with open esophagectomy.[7] Overall, the reported comparisons between MIE and open esophagectomy demonstrate MIE to be safe, with at least comparable outcomes in morbidity and mortality, and with some evidence to suggest better overall outcomes in terms of postoperative pulmonary complications, blood loss, and hospital stay. An important consideration regarding MIE for esophageal cancer is the adequacy of lymph node clearance as compared with the standard open esophagectomy. The 2 meta-analyses cited here have shown no difference in lymph node recovery rates between open esophagectomy and MIE.[5,6]

OPERATIVE TECHNIQUE

The operative technique used for a minimally invasive Ivor Lewis esophagectomy at Carolinas Medical Center is performed in 2 phases, beginning with laparoscopic mobilization of the stomach and dissection of the mediastinum from the abdomen. The technique is similar to that described by Bizekis and colleagues.[8] The operation is conducted by 2 surgical teams including fellows and residents, each led by an attending thoracic surgeon and gastrointestinal surgical oncologist.

Abdominal Phase

The patient is positioned supine on a split-leg table after intubation with a single-lumen endotracheal tube. The operation begins with diagnostic laparoscopy through an umbilical port to look for evidence of distant metastatic spread, especially for tumors of the gastroesophageal junction. If no signs of metastatic disease are noted, a hand port is placed between the umbilicus and xiphoid. Three 5-mm ports are placed in the left upper quadrant: the first lateral to the rectus, the second lateral to the first below the costal margin, and the third at the anterior axillary line.

The dissection is begun on entering the lesser sac though the gastrocolic omentum, avoiding injury to the right gastroepiploic artery. Lymph node tissue from around the left gastric artery is dissected and resected en bloc with the specimen. An endoscopic GIA stapler is used to divide the left gastric artery and coronary vein. The right gastric artery is preserved. The lower mediastinum is dissected with bipolar cautery. The dissection clears nodal tissue from the surfaces of the left pleura, aorta, pericardium, and right pleura, and removes this tissue in continuity with the specimen. A gastric conduit is fashioned using the endoscopic GIA stapler, which is used to divide the lesser curvature of the stomach between right and left gastric arteries. Pyloroplasty or pyloromyotomy is routinely performed via the hand port incision.

Three 19F drains are left in place via the trocar sites for drainage: one into the left pleura, one into the right pleura posterior to the conduit, and one in the right abdomen inferior to the lateral segment of the liver. Finally, a 10F jejunostomy feeding catheter is placed through the abdominal wall just lateral to the rectus muscle.

Thoracic Phase

The endotracheal tube is exchanged for a double-lumen tube, and the patient is positioned in the left lateral decubitus position. A total of 5 ports are placed in the chest: camera port anterior and inferior, operating port posterior and inferior, grasping port inferior to tip of scapula posteriorly, retraction port anterior and superior, and a suction port halfway between the 2 anterior ports.

The right lung is deflated and the lung retracted to visualize the esophagus. The inferior pulmonary ligament is incised, and the pleura anterior and posterior to the esophagus is incised. Dissection proceeds to the level of the azygos vein, which is divided using a vascular endoscopic stapler. The esophagus is divided when complete dissection is achieved, and the gastric conduit is brought into the chest with the lesser curvature staple line oriented to the patient's right. An anastomosis is created in the chest using a circular stapler. A flip-top stapler anvil affixed to a nasogastric tube (OrVil; Covidien, Norwalk, CT, USA) is passed through the mouth and the distal end of the tube brought through a fenestration in the esophageal staple line.[9,10] The superior end of the lesser-curve staple line is opened, and a 25-mm stapler inserted through the posterior-inferior thoracic port. The stapler head is inserted through the opening in the lesser curvature, and its spike brought out through the greater curvature of the gastric conduit. The stapler components are mated and fired. The opening in the lesser curvature is reapproximated with a GIA stapler.

Three-Stage Esophagectomy

If a 3-stage esophagectomy is required because of the extent of disease, the operation begins with laparoscopic mobilization of the stomach and dissection of the lower mediastinum from the abdomen. The patient is then positioned laterally, and the thoracic esophagus dissected. The patient is then repositioned supine and a cervical incision is made, the proximal esophagus circumferentially dissected and divided, and the gastric conduit passed from the abdomen to the chest. A cervical anastomosis is constructed with a linear stapler.

Transhiatal Esophagectomy

For patients with early-stage disease who do not need a mediastinal lymph node dissection, a transhiatal esophagectomy is performed using laparoscopic mobilization of the stomach and construction of a gastric conduit. The lower mediastinum is dissected using laparoscopic instruments. The dissection from below is completed using a hand inserted through the hand port. The specimen is removed after simultaneous dissection from the abdominal and cervical incisions. A cervical anastomosis is constructed with a linear stapler.

POSTOPERATIVE CARE

All patients are admitted to the surgical intensive care unit for postoperative monitoring, where they are cared for in coordination with a group of surgical intensivists who provide around-the-clock coverage. Central venous and arterial lines are placed by anesthesia before the operation and are used for invasive hemodynamic monitoring in the postoperative period. Swan-Ganz catheters are not routinely placed for monitoring purposes. To a varying degree patients are left intubated in the immediate postoperative period; those patients with adequate presurgical pulmonary function undergo attempted extubation immediately after the operation. Those patients left intubated are weaned from the ventilator expeditiously with the goal of extubation on postoperative day 1. Beginning on the day of surgery, tube feeds are started at via the jejunostomy tube. Patients are given standard perioperative antibiotics, proton pump inhibitors, and β blockade. For pain control, an epidural is placed before induction of anesthesia.

On the first postoperative day, patients are started on low molecular weight heparin and feeding via jejunostomy tube is initiated. Ambulation is encouraged and patients are asked to sit in a chair. Patients are assessed for ability to transfer to the surgical ward with the goal of transfer on the second postoperative day.

On postoperative day 4, patients undergo a standard esophagogram under fluoroscopy with water-soluble contrast to assess for anastomotic leak and emptying of the conduit. The epidural catheter is removed on postoperative day 5, along with the urinary catheter. On postoperative day 7, patients undergo computed tomographic (CT) esophagography to assess again for anastomotic leak. After a normal CT esophagogram, the pleural drains are removed. Patients are discharged with nocturnal tube feedings. The tube feedings are weaned over the next 4 to 6 weeks in an outpatient setting. When possible, discharge is planned for postoperative day 9.

OUTCOMES

A total of 32 patients underwent some variant of MIE. Two patients early in the authors' experience underwent a hybrid procedure with laparoscopic mobilization of the stomach followed by thoracotomy. Transthoracic Ivor Lewis esophagectomy with laparoscopy and thoracoscopy were performed in 28. A 3-phase esophagectomy was performed in 1 patient and laparoscopic transhiatal esophagectomy in 1. Indications for operation were adenocarcinoma in 27 patients, squamous cell carcinoma in 3, and benign stricture in 2. Conversion to laparotomy and thoracotomy was necessary in 1 patient due to extensive adhesive disease, and conversion to thoracotomy was necessary in 1 patient due to bleeding. The mean age was 58 (range 22–71) years. Mean intraoperative blood loss was 380 mL. Major complications occurred in

13 patients (42%), as shown in **Table 1**. Delayed complications occurred in 2 patients, one of whom developed delayed gastric emptying after a pyloromyotomy and underwent a laparoscopic pyloroplasty. Another patient who did not undergo a drainage procedure at the time of esophagectomy was treated with a laparoscopic pyloromyotomy.

Four patients developed anastomotic leaks. Two were treated conservatively with drainage of the chest and enteral nutrition via feeding jejunostomy. Two were treated via endoscopic stents, one of whom later developed an esophagobronchial fistula that required thoracotomy and muscle flap interposition.

For comparison, a group of historical controls was selected, consisting of 102 open esophagectomies performed in the authors' hospital and 3 affiliated hospitals within the metropolitan area between 1995 and 2009. The median hospital stay after open esophagectomy was 17 days and operative mortality, 8.9%.

Median hospital stay for patients treated with MIE was 10.5 days, which is significantly shorter than the median hospital stay of the authors' historical controls of open esophagectomy ($P<.0008$, Mantel-Hantzel). Although there was no mortality in this series of 32 MIEs compared with 8.9% among the 102 open operations, this difference was not statistically significant ($P = .11$, Fisher's exact test).

DISCUSSION

For a community cancer center, the decision to establish a program in complex gastrointestinal surgery such as esophageal resection is one that must weigh the demand for services of an uncommon neoplasm with an assessment of the available resources. The resources available in a community cancer center will also need to be assessed relative to the availability of esophageal cancer services at referral institutions, which may treat a larger volume of cases. Particularly with cancers of lower incidence such as esophageal cancers, the annual volume of esophageal resection cases becomes an important factor in this decision making. In this context, a brief discussion of the relationship between surgical volume and outcomes seems in order.

The association between surgical volume and outcomes has been well described in several articles with a variety of methodologies.[11,12] These studies have come to different conclusions regarding whether it is the volume of the surgeon[13] or the hospital that seems to drive better outcomes, and whether high volume in one particular procedure translates to better outcomes in other procedures at the same hospital.[14] Several studies have extended the original observations to include cancer

Table 1
Complications

Minor Complications	No. of Cases	Major Complications	No. of Cases
Delirium	5	Pneumonia	7
Transfusion	4	Reintubation	5
Stricture requiring dilation	4	Acute respiratory distress syndrome	4
Jejunostomy tube leakage	3	Anastomotic leak	4
Jejunostomy tube dislodged	1	Delayed gastric emptying	2
Deep venous thrombosis	1	Tracheostomy	2
Wound infection	1	Pulmonary embolism	1
		Recurrent laryngeal nerve palsy	1
		Stroke	1
		Chylothorax	1

surgery.[15] A collective review[16] concluded that surgeon volume and specialization are more strongly associated with outcomes than hospital volume. A similar review of cancer surgery[17] found a consistent relationship between volume and outcome, but could not distinguish the effect of hospital volume from surgical volume. Of note, one-third of the 101 publications reviewed show no effect of volume on outcome.

Several studies have examined the relationship between volume and outcome in esophageal surgery, with similar findings.[18–25]

Surgical volume has become, in many cases, the primary end point in predicting quality of outcomes. Volume is an attractive surrogate for other measures such as operative mortality or overall survival, as it is easy to measure and does not suffer from the statistical hazards of evaluation of mortality in small sample sizes.[26]

Based on these observations, recommendations have been made that patients undergoing complex cancer surgery be referred to high-volume institutions. Calculations have been generated about how many lives might be saved if practice patterns were changed in this way.[27,28] Since the initial studies in the 1980s describing the relationship between volume and outcomes, practice patterns have evolved such that complex cancer surgery has been shifted to centers with higher volume.[29,30]

Few empirical data exist regarding the effects of selective referral of esophageal resections to high-volume centers. One example is a network of 11 hospitals in western Netherlands, who agreed to direct referrals to high-volume centers within their network. Subsequent to this agreement, mortality declined within their system. When the later time period was examined, however, equal numbers of patients underwent esophagectomies in high-volume and low-volume hospitals, with shorter hospital stay in the high-volume hospitals, but equal mortality in the two hospital groups. By contrast, similar efforts of centralization of esophageal cancer care in Scotland did not result in significant reduction in operative mortality, but did lead to longer delays in treatment.[31]

In a country the size of the United States, by contrast, patient travel time to a high-volume center becomes an important consideration. The centralization of esophageal resections in western Netherlands, for example, was made easier by a maximum distance of 30 miles between the hospitals. By contrast, residents in the Southern United States are estimated to have a median travel time of more than 2 hours to a National Cancer Institute (NCI)-designated cancer center, but less than 45 minutes to care at an academic medical center.[32] Calculations have shown that depending on where the volume threshold for esophageal resection is set, if selective referral to high-volume centers were to occur, 80% of patients would need to change to high-volume centers with significant increases in travel time.[33] The provision of access to cancer care, especially in rural areas, demands that efforts be made to provide high-quality cancer care close to home, suggesting a critical role for the community cancer center.

While there is an intuitive appeal to the concept that "practice makes perfect," other data suggest that the simple equation of high volume with better outcomes may be overly simplistic. The Veterans Affairs NSQIP study, with careful risk stratification, found no difference between high-volume and low-volume hospitals.[34] Data from the National Inpatient Study suggest that the volume-outcome curve is actually U-shaped, with mortality increasing at very high-volume institutions.[35] Several low-volume centers have reported their outcomes after complex gastrointestinal cancer surgery, with outcomes equivalent to high-volume centers.[36–38] These latter studies likely suffer from some selection bias, as low-volume centers with inferior outcomes may be less likely to publish their results. Nonetheless, these factors together suggest that complex gastrointestinal cancer surgery is feasible in lower-volume centers.

The determinants of high-quality esophageal surgery apart from surgical volume have been less well studied, but some studies suggest mechanisms by which volume is related to outcomes. Surgeons' specialty training appears to be related to outcomes, with fellowship specialty training being associated with better outcomes.[39,40] Outcomes at NCI-designated cancer centers appear to be better than outcomes at hospitals with similar volumes, suggesting that factors other than volume may be important.[41] NCI-designated cancer centers, for instance, are demonstrated to have higher ratios of nurses to patients. A review of outcomes after gastrectomy suggests that nurse staffing and the number of intensive care unit beds are associated with better outcomes.[42]

Although the surgical outcomes are no doubt affected by what transpires within the operating room, there is evidence that mortality outcomes are influenced by the quality of perioperative care as well. Some studies suggest that although the incidence of certain complications tends to have small differences between hospitals with low and high mortality rates, patients are more likely to survive those complications at low-mortality hospitals.[43,44] The so-called "failure to rescue" is lower in these hospitals, and is likely influenced by a host of resources for perioperative care such as nurse training, and the support of specialists in intensive care, diagnostic radiology, interventional radiology, and gastroenterology.

SUMMARY

The authors' current average volume of 13 esophageal resections per year could best be characterized as moderate to high. This average annual volume is certainly less than some centers, but is also greater than many of the suggested volume thresholds, including that set by the Leapfrog group. Data from the National Inpatient Sample would suggest at as of 2006, only 12.4% of hospitals had esophagectomy volumes greater than 13 per year.[35]

Although the series is small, outcomes of mortality and hospital length of stay are improved compared with historical controls in the authors' own hospital system and compare favorably with national norms. Hospitals in the National Inpatient Study had a 7% operative mortality for esophagectomy in 2006.[35]

The authors' anecdotal experience is that surgical volume increased after implementation of a program in MIE, rather than before. One of the key elements of this program is the collaboration between specialist surgeons in thoracic surgery and gastrointestinal surgical oncology. The authors also benefit from strong institutional support and resources including full-time intensivist coverage in the surgical intensive care unit, an outpatient nutritionist in the cancer center, a fellowship-trained gastrointestinal pathologist, and a dedicated surgical team of nurses and anesthetists.

The authors' experience would suggest that a community hospital with a committed team and sufficient resources can provide high-quality care for patients with esophageal cancer. Although esophageal cancer remains an uncommon neoplasm, adenocarcinoma of the distal esophagus is rapidly increasing in incidence,[45] suggesting that demand for esophageal resection will increase in the future. This scenario would suggest that despite current trends for the increased centralization of esophageal cancer care, a critical role still exists for community cancer centers in the care of these patients.

REFERENCES

1. Schoppmann SF, Prager G, Langer F, et al. Fifty-five minimally invasive esophagectomies: a single centre experience. Anticancer Res 2009;29(7):2719–25.

2. Cuschieri A, Shimi S, Banting S. Endoscopic oesophagectomy through a right thoracoscopic approach. J R Coll Surg Edinb 1992;37(1):7–11.

3. Dallemagne B. Endoscopic approaches to oesophageal disease. Baillieres Clin Gastroenterol 1993;7(4):795–822.

4. Smithers BM. Minimally invasive esophagectomy: an overview. Expert Rev Gastroenterol Hepatol 2010;4(1):91–9.

5. Nagpal K, Ahmed K, Vats A, et al. Is minimally invasive surgery beneficial in the management of esophageal cancer? A meta-analysis. Surg Endosc 2010;24(7): 1621–9.

6. Sgourakis G, Gockel I, Radtke A, et al. Minimally invasive versus open esophagectomy: meta-analysis of outcomes. Dig Dis Sci 2010;55(11):3031–40.

7. Lazzarino AI, Nagpal K, Bottle A, et al. Open versus minimally invasive esophagectomy: trends of utilization and associated outcomes in England. Ann Surg 2010;252(2):292–8.

8. Bizekis C, Kent MS, Luketich JD, et al. Initial experience with minimally invasive Ivor Lewis esophagectomy. Ann Thorac Surg 2006;82(2):402–6.

9. Matthews BD, Sing RF, DeLegge MH, et al. Initial results with a stapled gastrojejunostomy for the laparoscopic isolated roux-en-Y gastric bypass. Am J Surg 2000;179(6):476–81.

10. Nguyen TN, Hinojosa MW, Smith BR, et al. Thoracoscopic construction of an intrathoracic esophagogastric anastomosis using a circular stapler: transoral placement of the anvil. Ann Thorac Surg 2008;86(3):989–92.

11. Luft HS, Bunker JP, Enthoven AC. Should operations be regionalized? The empirical relation between surgical volume and mortality. N Engl J Med 1979;301(25): 1364–9.

12. Birkmeyer JD, Siewers AE, Finlayson EV, et al. Hospital volume and surgical mortality in the United States. N Engl J Med 2002;346(15):1128–37.

13. Birkmeyer JD, Stukel TA, Siewers AE, et al. Surgeon volume and operative mortality in the United States. N Engl J Med 2003;349(22):2117–27.

14. Urbach DR, Baxter NN. Does it matter what a hospital is "high volume" for? Specificity of hospital volume-outcome associations for surgical procedures: analysis of administrative data. BMJ 2004;328(7442):737–40.

15. Finlayson EV, Goodney PP, Birkmeyer JD. Hospital volume and operative mortality in cancer surgery: a national study. Arch Surg 2003;138(7):721–5.

16. Chowdhury MM, Dagash H, Pierro A. A systematic review of the impact of volume of surgery and specialization on patient outcome. Br J Surg 2007;94(2):145–61.

17. Gruen RL, Pitt V, Green S, et al. The effect of provider case volume on cancer mortality: systematic review and meta-analysis. CA Cancer J Clin 2009;59(3): 192–211.

18. Leigh Y, Goldacre M, McCulloch P. Surgical specialty, surgical unit volume and mortality after oesophageal cancer surgery. Eur J Surg Oncol 2009;35(8): 820–5.

19. Metzger R, Bollschweiler E, Vallbohmer D, et al. High volume centers for esophagectomy: what is the number needed to achieve low postoperative mortality? Dis Esophagus 2004;17(4):310–4.

20. Dimick JB, Cattaneo SM, Lipsett PA, et al. Hospital volume is related to clinical and economic outcomes of esophageal resection in Maryland. Ann Thorac Surg 2001;72(2):334–9.

21. Ra J, Paulson EC, Kucharczuk J, et al. Postoperative mortality after esophagectomy for cancer: development of a preoperative risk prediction model. Ann Surg Oncol 2008;15(6):1577–84.

22. Lauder CI, Marlow NE, Maddern GJ, et al. Systematic review of the impact of volume of oesophagectomy on patient outcome. ANZ J Surg 2010;80(5): 317–23.
23. Reavis KM, Smith BR, Hinojosa MW, et al. Outcomes of esophagectomy at academic centers: an association between volume and outcome. Am Surg 2008;74(10):939–43.
24. Rodgers M, Jobe BA, O'Rourke RW, et al. Case volume as a predictor of inpatient mortality after esophagectomy. Arch Surg 2007;142(9):829–39.
25. Boudourakis LD, Wang TS, Roman SA, et al. Evolution of the surgeon-volume, patient-outcome relationship. Ann Surg 2009;250(1):159–65.
26. Dimick JB, Welch HG, Birkmeyer JD. Surgical mortality as an indicator of hospital quality: the problem with small sample size. JAMA 2004;292(7):847–51.
27. Birkmeyer JD, Dimick JB. Potential benefits of the new Leapfrog standards: effect of process and outcomes measures. Surgery 2004;135(6):569–75.
28. Birkmeyer JD, Finlayson EV, Birkmeyer CM. Volume standards for high-risk surgical procedures: potential benefits of the Leapfrog initiative. Surgery 2001; 130(3):415–22.
29. Stitzenberg KB, Sigurdson ER, Egleston BL, et al. Centralization of cancer surgery: implications for patient access to optimal care. J Clin Oncol 2009; 27(28):4671–8.
30. Ho V, Heslin MJ, Yun H, et al. Trends in hospital and surgeon volume and operative mortality for cancer surgery. Ann Surg Oncol 2006;13(6):851–8.
31. Milne AA, Skinner J, Browning G. Centralisation of oesophageal cancer services; the view from the periphery. J R Coll Surg Edinb 2000;45(3):164–7.
32. Onega T, Duell EJ, Shi X, et al. Geographic access to cancer care in the U.S. Cancer 2008;112(4):909–18.
33. Birkmeyer JD, Siewers AE, Marth NJ, et al. Regionalization of high-risk surgery and implications for patient travel times. JAMA 2003;290(20):2703–8.
34. Khuri SF, Daley J, Henderson W, et al. Relation of surgical volume to outcome in eight common operations: results from the VA National Surgical Quality Improvement Program. Ann Surg 1999;230(3):414–29.
35. Kohn GP, Galanko JA, Meyers MO, et al. National trends in esophageal surgery— are outcomes as good as we believe? J Gastrointest Surg 2009;13(11):1900–10.
36. Reasbeck PG. Treatment of oesophageal carcinoma at a small rural hospital. J R Coll Surg Edinb 1998;43(5):314–7.
37. Courrech Staal EF, van CF, Cats A, et al. Outcome of low-volume surgery for esophageal cancer in a high-volume referral center. Ann Surg Oncol 2009; 16(12):3219–26.
38. Guzzo MH, Landercasper J, Boyd WC, et al. Outcomes of complex gastrointestinal procedures performed in a community hospital. WMJ 2005;104(6):30–4.
39. Dimick JB, Goodney PP, Orringer MB, et al. Specialty training and mortality after esophageal cancer resection. Ann Thorac Surg 2005;80(1):282–6.
40. Schipper PH, Diggs BS, Ungerleider RM, et al. The influence of surgeon specialty on outcomes in general thoracic surgery: a national sample 1996 to 2005. Ann Thorac Surg 2009;88(5):1566–72.
41. Birkmeyer NJ, Goodney PP, Stukel TA, et al. Do cancer centers designated by the National Cancer Institute have better surgical outcomes? Cancer 2005;103(3): 435–41.
42. Smith DL, Elting LS, Learn PA, et al. Factors influencing the volume-outcome relationship in gastrectomies: a population-based study. Ann Surg Oncol 2007;14(6): 1846–52.

43. Ghaferi AA, Osborne NH, Birkmeyer JD, et al. Hospital characteristics associated with failure to rescue from complications after pancreatectomy. J Am Coll Surg 2010;211(3):325–30.
44. Ghaferi AA, Birkmeyer JD, Dimick JB. Complications, failure to rescue, and mortality with major inpatient surgery in Medicare patients. Ann Surg 2009; 250(6):1029–34.
45. Brown LM, Devesa SS, Chow WH. Incidence of adenocarcinoma of the esophagus among white Americans by sex, stage, and age. J Natl Cancer Inst 2008; 100(16):1184–7.

Cancer Immunotherapy

Richard L. White Jr, MD[a],*, Asim Amin, MD, PhD[b]

KEYWORDS

• Immunotherapy • Cancer • Vaccine • Cytokines

On April 29, 2010, the US Food and Drug Administration (FDA) approved sipuleucel-T (Provenge) for the treatment of men with advanced, hormonally refractive, prostate cancer. With this, the notion of vaccines for the treatment of advanced cancer became a reality for individuals suffering from advanced prostate cancer. This breakthrough comes a century after the recognition by Coley that immunologic events, specifically infections, could result in regression of established cancer.[1] Over the last century, the relationship between the immune system and the tumor environment has been explored on multiple levels with efforts to enhance immunity, tumor recognition, or both. These efforts are now making their way into the community with a number of immunologic agents approved by the FDA for ongoing use. For the purposes of this article, the authors focus on solid tumors and explore these immunologic approaches including cytokines, vaccines, antibody-based therapy, and cellular therapies—many of which are currently or will become common fare in community cancer programs.

CYTOKINES

The administration of high-dose, bolus interleukin (IL)-2 has consistently led to prolonged durable responses in patients with metastatic melanoma and kidney cancer. The demonstration by Rosenberg and colleagues[2,3] of the efficacy of an immune modulating cytokine on established tumor clearly demonstrated the potential of immune-based therapies.

No funding support was received for this work.

Conflicts of interest: Dr White is a member of the speakers bureau for Schering Plough.

Dr Amin is on the speakers bureau and is a consultant for Novartis. In addition, Dr Amin is a consultant for Argos. He is a clinical investigator for the Abbot, Argos, BMS, AB science, and Altor studies.

[a] Division of Surgical Oncology, Carolinas Medical Center, Blumenthal Cancer Center, 1025 Morehead Medical Drive, Suite 600, Charlotte, NC 28204, USA

[b] Department of Medicine, Carolinas Medical Center, Blumenthal Cancer Center, 1025 Morehead Medical Drive, Charlotte, NC 28204, USA

* Corresponding author.

E-mail address: Richard.White@carolinashealthcare.org

IL-2 is a 15.5 kD glycoprotein hormone with pluripotent immunomodulating properties including T cell activation[4] that leads to downstream cascade and the release of other cytokines including IL-1, tumor necrosis factor, interferon-γ, IL-6, and lymphotoxin. These other cytokines may also contribute to the efficacy and side effects of IL-2 therapy and decrease after IL-2 treatment is completed.[5]

Dose escalation trials were begun in the 1980s in patients with a variety of cancers. In a series of 25 patients, IL-2 resulted in significant responses in patients with advanced renal cell cancer (RCC) and in patients with refractory metastatic melanoma.[3] Patients with metastatic RCC have historically had a median survival of 12 months and patients with melanoma 4 to 12 months.[6] Large trials of patients with metastatic melanoma have shown a consistent response rate of 12% to 16%, with a 6% complete response rate.[7,8] Trials of patients with refractory RCC have repeatedly demonstrated a response rate of 14% to 23% with 4% to 8% having a complete response.[8–10] These responses have been remarkably durable, especially in patients who achieve a complete response. In both groups of patients, the median survival has not been reached. Work from the Cytokine Working Group and the authors' data over the last decade have confirmed these findings.

The concern regarding the use of IL-2 stems from the significant toxicities associated with the administration of the high-dose regimen (720,000 IU/kg or 600,000 IU/kg intravenously every 8 hours). Most patients receive 6 to 10 doses in a cycle usually stopping due to dose-limiting toxicities or fatigue. Patients then return in 7 to 14 days for another cycle of therapy. If they have stable or responding disease, two additional cycles (also referred to as a course) are offered. A third course is usually limited to patients who have tolerated the treatment relatively well and have ongoing shrinkage of disease. This dosing schedule has been associated with a well described capillary leak phenomenon that routinely causes oliguria, mild hypoxemia, generalized edema, and hypotension.[7,11] The expected toxicities are shown in **Table 1**. Although these toxicities require hospitalization and dedicated support, they can be well

Table 1
Expected toxicities with IL-2 treatment

System	Toxicities	Percent IL-2 Courses in Which Grade 3 or 4 Toxicity Occurred N = 288
Cardiovascular	Atrial or ventricular arrhythmias	12.2
—	Hypotension requiring pressors	38.2
Fatigue	Difficulty performing some activities	1.4
GI	Nausea and vomiting (severe)	1.7
—	Diarrhea (severe)	1.0
Hematologic	Low platelet count (<50,000)	9.7
	Low white blood count (<1,000)	0.7
Neurologic	Anxiety or depression (severe)	1.4
—	Confusion	2.4
Pulmonary	Shortness of breath (severe)	1.0
Renal	Elevated creatinine	0.35
—	Peripheral edema	0.7
—	Poor urine output	6.3

Data from Carolinas Medical Center, Charlotte, NC.

managed with limited mortality.[8] In our community teaching hospital, we have treated 196 patients with high-dose IL-2, administering 599 cycles of treatment with only one treatment-associated death.

Significant responses can be achieved in patients with established metastases (**Figs. 1** and **2**). **Fig. 3** displays the survival curves of patients responding to IL-2 therapy.[8] **Table 2** details the response rates and durability of the responses. Based on the remarkable durability of the responses and the impact on a patient with a complete response, IL-2 was approved by the FDA in 1992 for use in patients with metastatic renal cell cancer and in 1998 for patients with advanced melanoma.

Given the toxicities and the relatively limited response rate, there have been extensive efforts to define the optimal candidate for IL-2 therapy. With the exception of pretreatment performance status, no consistent reproducible pattern has been observed.[9,11] Clearly, higher response rates and more durable responses are observed in individuals with subcutaneous, nodal, and lung disease compared with responses in patients with liver, bone, and brain metastases.[7]

Efforts have been made to reduce toxicity by reducing the dose of IL-2. Yang and colleagues[12] reported on the use of low-dose IL-2 (72,000 IU/kg) in patients with advanced kidney cancer. Although there were substantially fewer toxicities, there was no difference in treatment mortality, and the response rate was 13% compared with 21% for high-dose IL-2. Lower doses of IL-2 in patients with metastatic melanoma have shown little efficacy.

Given the remarkable longevity of patients achieving significant partial or complete responses to IL-2 and given that the toxicities can be well managed and are of very limited duration (typically 4–6 days during a course of therapy), the authors believe that all eligible patients with advanced melanoma and renal cancer should be offered IL-2.

IL-2 Plus Vaccine

IL-2 for injection should be restricted to patients with normal cardiac and pulmonary function. Extreme caution is needed in patients with a normal thallium stress test and pulmonary function test who have a history of cardiac or pulmonary disease.

IL-2 should be administered in a hospital under the supervision of a physician experienced in using anticancer agents. An intensive care facility and cardiopulmonary specialists must be available.

IL-2 can cause capillary leak syndrome (CLS; loss of vascular tone and extravasation of plasma proteins and fluid into the extravascular space). CLS can cause hypotension and reduced organ perfusion, which can cause death, cardiac arrhythmias (supraventricular and ventricular), angina, myocardial infarction, respiratory

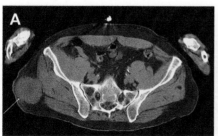
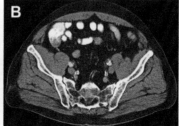

Fig. 1. Response of metastatic melanoma of the subcutaneous tissues (*arrow*) overlying the pelvis before (*A*) and after (*B*) high-dose IL-2 treatment.

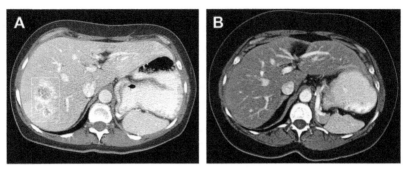

Fig. 2. Response of metastatic renal cell cancer lesions (*box*) to the liver before (*A*) and after (*B*) high-dose IL-2 treatment.

insufficiency requiring intubation, gastrointestinal bleeding or infarction, renal insufficiency, edema, and mental status changes.

IL-2 treatment can impair neutrophil function and cause disseminated infection, including sepsis and bacterial endocarditis. Consequently, preexisting bacterial infections must be treated before IL-2 treatment. Patients with indwelling central lines are at risk for infection with gram-positive microorganisms. Antibiotic prophylaxis with oxacillin, nafcillin, ciprofloxacin, or vancomycin may reduce the incidence of staphylococcal infections.

IL-2 administration should be withheld in patients developing moderate-to-severe lethargy or somnolence; continued administration can result in coma.[13]

Given the clinical activity of IL-2, many efforts have been made to augment its efficacy. Additionally, it has been demonstrated that IL-2 can serve as a powerful immunologic adjuvant. Gp100: 209–217 (210M), a peptide derived from a lineage-restricted melanoma antigen enhanced to augment HLA-A2.1 binding, has been shown to stimulate T cell responses in vitro and in vivo.[14] Early work at the National Cancer Institute

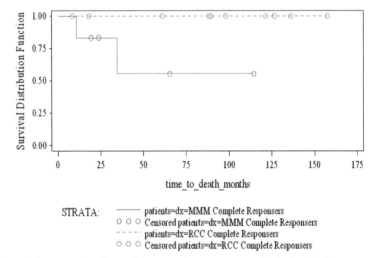

Fig. 3. Survival curves of patients with a complete response to high-dose IL-2 treatment at Carolinas Medical Center. dx, diagnosis; MMM, metastatic melanoma; RCC, renal cell carcinoma.

Table 2
Complete and partial responses to high-dose IL-2 treatment

Treatment Date	Renal Cell Cancer				Melanoma			
	Number of Patients Treated	Response Rate (CR + PR) No. (%)	Ongoing Responses No. (%)	Duration of All Responses (Months)[a]	Number of Patients Treated	Response Rate (CR + PR) No. (%)	Ongoing Responses No. (%)	Duration of All Responses (Months)[a]
1998 through 2009	86	23 (26.7) [CR = 6 (7%) PR = 17 (19.8%)]	7 (8.1)	CR: 98+, 89+, 61+, 23, 18+, 8+ PR: 58+, 24, 23+, 22, 19, 17, 16, 15, 13, 11, 11, 10, 9, 7, 6, 5, 3	92	13 (14.1) [CR = 4 (4.3%) PR = 9 (9.8%)]	7 (7.6%)	CR: 114+, 43, 24+, 19+ PR: 73+, 51+, 28+, 24+, 12, 8, 6, 5, 4

Abbreviations: CR, complete response; PR, partial response.
[a] Duration of response on 12/31/2009 for patients completing IL-2 treatment; + indicates ongoing response.
Data from Carolinas Medical Center, Charlotte, NC.

Surgery Branch that combined 210M with high-dose, bolus IL-2 showed a dramatic 42% response rate (vs historical response rate with IL-2 alone of 16%).[15]

The Cytokine Working Group preformed three phase II trails from 1998 to 2003 examining 131 HLA A2-positive patients using varying schedules. Response rates of 23% (trial 1), 12.5% (trial 2), and 12.8% (trial 3) were observed. The investigators concluded that these trials "did not demonstrate the promising clinical activity" previously noted.[16]

Schwartzentruber and colleagues[17] have completed a phase III randomized trial comparing high-dose IL-2 with IL-2 plus gp100. The response rate in the group receiving vaccine was significantly better than with IL-2 alone (22.1% vs 9.7%, $P = .02$) as was progression-free survival (2.9 months vs 1.6 months, $P = .008$). This is the first trial demonstrating a clinical benefit of vaccination in patients with melanoma.

Interferon

With the demonstration of cytokine activity in patients with advanced cancer, studies of the use of cytokines have been expanded to patients with earlier stages. Interferon-α administered to patients with advanced melanoma led to substantive responses[18]; however, few of these have been durable. Given the activity, however, efforts began in earnest to test interferons in the adjuvant setting. Kirkwood and Ernstoff[19] initiated the Eastern Cooperative Oncology Group (ECOG) Trial E1684, which effectively administered interferon at a the maximum tolerated dose given for 4 weeks intravenously (20 MU/m^2 daily for 5 days) followed by a maintenance dose (10 MU/subcutaneously 3 times/week) for another 48 weeks. In 287 high-risk melanoma patients with primarily stage III disease, there was improvement in both relapse-free and overall survival (relapse-free survival: observation = 0.98 years, treatment = 1.72 years, $P = .0023$; overall survival: observation = 2.78 years, treatment = 3.82 years, $P = .0237$).[19] Based on these data, the FDA approved the use of interferon in patients at high risk of melanoma recurrence.

Two subsequent trials have been performed using this regimen. E1690 compared the approved dose with a lower dose regimen (3 MU/d 3 times per week for 2 years) or observation.[20] In this trial, more patients with stage II disease were enrolled than in the 1684 trial. Once again a relapse-free survival benefit was noted, yet the overall survival was the same. Further retrospective analysis demonstrated that 31% of patients in the observation arm received interferon after relapse.[20] E1694 compared high-dose interferon with a GM2 ganglioside melanoma antigen conjugated to keyhole limpet hemocyanin and administered with QS-21 (a nonspecific immune adjuvant) given over 2 years.[21] Once again, a relapse-free survival benefit was observed; however, this trial was stopped prematurely due to significant differences in overall survival between the two arms. A meta-analysis of interferon as a treatment strategy has been performed demonstrating an improvement in disease-free survival (DFS) (hazard ratio [HR] for recurrence 0.82, $P<.001$) and an improvement in overall survival (HR for death 0.89, $P = .002$).[22]

The toxicities associated with the administration of the approved regimen and the dosing schedules for interferon have led to the investigation of potentially less toxic longer acting preparations. The European Organisation for Research and Treatment of Cancer (EORTC) trial 18991 assessed the utility of pegylated interferon alfa-2b given subcutaneously at 6 μg/kg per week for 8 weeks then 3 μg/kg per week for an intended duration of 5 years in high-risk patients with resected stage III melanoma.[23] The 4-year recurrence-free survival was 45.6% in the interferon group compared with 38.9% in the observation arm (HR 0.82, $P = .01$, n = 1256 patients). There was no benefit to overall survival. Forty percent of patients in the interferon group had grade 3 toxicities versus 10% in the observation group. The FDA is currently considering approval of pegylated interferon for use in the United States.

Given the reported demonstration of the impact of interferon on the natural history of melanoma, the authors recommend consideration in all eligible patients. Toxicities are notable but can be mitigated. In centers with experience, the majority of patients can complete a year of therapy.[21]

Studies to examine the efficacy of other cytokines have been met with limited success, with none having been approved for therapy.

VACCINES

The notion of a vaccine for cancer therapy is very attractive. The administration of a compound with limited toxicity that can induce an immunologic tumor response, much in the same way as viruses are approached, seems straightforward. Investigators have identified tumor antigens (eg, MART 1, MAGE-3 for melanoma, prostatic acid phosphatase [PAP], and prostate-specific membrane antigen in prostate cancer). Immune responses to these antigens can be generated[24] and can be augmented with a variety of compounds (eg, granulocyte-macrophage colony-stimulating factor [GM-CSF],[25] IL-23[26]). The issue has been how and when to use these agents and in what form. Vaccines prepared from cell lysates, peptides, and augmented cell lysates have been tested in clinical trials. Inherent to the notion of a vaccine is the interplay between antigen and immune system. Of necessity, the antigens must be weakly antigenic, otherwise the immune system would rapidly identify and destroy the malignant cells. Equally as important is the recognition of the antigen by the immune system, most notably cytotoxic T lymphocytes (CTLs). In order for the CTLs to recognize antigens, the antigen must first be presented by an APC. The most powerful of these are dendritic cells so named because of their dendrites that increase surface area allowing for interaction with many CTLs. APCs internalize antigens present in the environment, process them, and present peptides in the context of major histocompatibility complexes (MHCs). This process in the context of costimulatory molecules leads to the activation of CTLs, which can then recognize antigens. CTLs cannot recognize antigens independently and are dependant on the presentation of peptides in the context of MHC on the surface of the APC. These costimulatory molecules (eg, B7-1, ICAM 1, LFA 3) function as a second signal necessary for immune (CTL) activation. Using these necessary ingredients for a robust immune activation has led to a plethora of vaccine strategies.

A review of the National Cancer Institute Surgery Branch experience with vaccines in 440 patients with advanced cancer demonstrated a response rate of 2.6%, commensurate with reports by others.[24] This very low response rate in established tumors may be considered irrelevant; established viral infections are not treated with vaccinations with the expectation of resolution of the ongoing illness.

On this basis, investigators have looked to situations where there is little tumor burden in patients with malignancies with identifiable tumor antigens. Melanoma and prostate cancer have met these requirements. In addition, both patient populations tend to have long periods when they are symptom free.

Sipuleucel-T (Provenge)

Sipuleucel-T is an autologous APC-based vaccine that is produced by pulsing APCs harvested from the patient in vitro with PA2024, a recombinant fusion protein of human PAP and GM-CSF. Five hundred twelve patients were enrolled in the Immunotherapy for Prostate Adenocarcinoma Treatment (IMPACT) trial that led to recent FDA approval.[27] Patients with asymptomatic or minimally symptomatic castration-resistant, prostate cancer were enrolled. All patients had a Gleason score of 7 or lower at the outset of the study; but, after gaining further evidence, men with higher scores were enrolled. Patients had to have a prostate-specific antigen (PSA) of 5 ng per ml or higher, progressive disease based on rising PSA or imaging studies, and a good performance status (ECOG 0 or 1). Patients were excluded if they had visceral metastases, long bone fractures, recent steroid exposure or radiation, chemotherapy within 3 months, prior therapy with more than two chemotherapy regimens, or spinal cord compression. Patients were randomized in a 2:1 ratio to receive either sipuleucel-T or placebo every 2 weeks for a total of three infusions. The treatment consisted of three standard leukapheresis procedures of 1.5 to 2 times the patients estimated blood volume at weeks 0, 2, and 4. Each of these was then followed 3 days later by infusion of sipuleucel-T or placebo cells. The cells were prepared centrally. The APCs were cultured for 36 to 44 hours with PA2024. Placebo cells were prepared without PA2024. PA2024 consists of a PAP, a prostate tumor antigen that is fused to GM-CSF, an immunostimulant. The cells were administered over 60 minutes after pretreatment of the patient with acetaminophen and an antihistamine. Response was monitored with CT scans, bone scan, and PSA. At the time of progression, the patient was unblinded and could be treated at the physician's discretion, including cryopreserved cells treated in the same fashion as sipuleucel-T. Five hundred twelve patients were enrolled; 341 received sipuleucel-T and 171 placebo. Median time from first infusion to the third infusion was 28 days. The median age was 71 years; 53.9% had had prostate radiation and 35.2% radical prostatectomy. The median follow-up was 34.1 months; median survival was 25.8 months in the sipuleucel-T group versus 21.7 months in the placebo group. The unadjusted HR for death was 0.77 (95% CI 0.61–0.98), a relative reduction of 23% ($P = .02$). The estimated 36-month survival after randomization was 31.7% in the sipuleucel-T group and 23.0% in the placebo group. One of the 341 patients in the sipuleucel-T group had a partial tumor response and 3% had a 50% or greater reduction in PSA. There was no difference in the time to progression (14.6 weeks in the sipuleucel-T cohort vs 14.4 weeks in the placebo group, $P = .63$, HR 0.95). No autoimmune phenomena were noted, and no patient suffered anaphylaxis. In short, the patients lived longer without a tumor response. The investigators suggest that these effects "may be due to the delayed onset of anti-tumor responses after active immunotherapy."

Active (stimulating a host tumor response) specific (inciting tumor recognition) immunotherapy approaches are evolving including PROSTVAC-VF, a vaccine composed of two recombinant viral vectors each encoding genes for PSA and three immunostimulatory molecules (B7.1, ICAM-1, and LFA-3). As seen with sipuleucel-T, there was an improvement in median survival (8.5 months) in the absence of progression-free survival.[28] Further trials are underway.

Allovectin-7

Allovectin-7 contains the plasmid DNA (pDNA) VCL-1005 encoding human leukocyte antigen B7 (HLA-B7) heavy chain and B2-microglobulin proteins. This plasmid DNA can be administered by intralesional injection.[29] In patients who are HLA-B7-negative, there is evidence of a response against the now expressed HLA-B7. In addition, the vaccine appears to upregulate or restore expression of MHC I molecules. The final proposed mechanism is predicated on an inflammatory response to the pDNA-lipid vaccine complex.

In a phase 2 trial of Allovectin-7 injection in 127 patients with either stage IV or unresectable stage III melanoma limited to skin, subcutaneous tissue, lymph nodes, or lung. Four patients (3.1%) had a complete response, and 11 (8.7%) had a partial response.[29] The median duration of response was 13.8 months (range, 6.0 to 66.2 + months); the median survival was 18.8 months, with 13 of 15 responders alive at the time of database lock. Nineteen percent of patients with more than one lesion identified at baseline (19 of 102) had a noninjected lesion response (10 regional and 9 systemic).[29] Comparison of Allovectin-7 plus dacarbazine versus dacarbazine alone showed no difference in response rate (13.2% vs 11.6%) or median survival (10.75 months vs 9.24 months).[30]

Ongoing trials compare Allovectin-7 alone to either DTIC or temozolomide in chemotherapy-naïve, stage III or IV melanoma patients.

Cellular Vaccines

Tumor cells, obtained from operative specimens or from cultivated cell lines of a specific patient and subsequently treated to prevent replication, can be used to create autologous tumor cell vaccines. The appeal of this approach is that the patient is exposed to all possible tumor antigens. These vaccines are usually administered with an immune adjuvant to create an inflammatory environment. An example of this is M-Vax, which is being used in a phase III trial.

Tumor is harvested from the patient and treated with dinitrophenol (DNP) to augment immune recognition. Berd and colleagues[31,32] at Thomas Jefferson Medical Center have demonstrated improved disease-free and overall survival compared with historical controls in patients with resected stage III melanoma. Patients enrolled in this trial will undergo vaccination with M-Vax (autologous DNP modified tumor cells) followed by cyclophosphamide and then 6 weekly doses of M-Vax administered with bacillus of Calmette and Guérin (BCG). Following vaccine, these patients will receive low doses of IL-2. Patients in the control group will receive a placebo vaccine and the regimen described above.[33] The end point is response rate in patients with stage IV melanoma.

Allogeneic Vaccines

Tumor-based vaccines in which the cells are derived from different patients are termed allogeneic. Typically, these vaccines are comprised of cells derived from multiple cell lines in an effort to provide exposure to multiple cancer antigens. Perhaps the most studied of these vaccines is Canvaxin, initially developed by Dr Donald Morton and his colleagues at the John Wayne Cancer Institute, and Melacine developed by Dr Malcolm Mitchell.

Mitchell and colleagues[34] used two cell lines, mechanically lysed the cells, and administered them with the adjuvant DETOX (detoxified Freund's adjuvant) and named this Melacine. In initial phase I trials, clinical responses occurred in 5 of 17 patients. Responders were noted to have circulatory cytotoxic T cell precursors. Further investigation revealed an association between response and the HLA alleles A2, B12, and C3. Based on this preliminary work, the Southwest Oncology Group performed a randomized trial in patients with resected disease.[35] Six hundred ninety-nine patients with intermediate thickness (1.5–4.0 mm), node-negative melanoma were randomized to vaccine for 2 years or observation. At a median follow-up of 5.6 years, there were 107 recurrences or deaths in the 300 patients receiving vaccine versus 114 among the 300 observation patients (HR 0.92; $p_2 = 0.51$).

Five-year estimated, DFS rates were 65% for the vaccine arm and 63% for the observation patients. At the time of its publication, this was the largest randomized, controlled trial of vaccine therapy for human cancer ever reported. The major flaw of this trial is noteworthy: it was powered to detect a 50% increase in median relapse-free survival (a very unlikely event). Of interest, a subset analysis based on MHC class I antigen expression demonstrated improved relapse-free survival in patients with HLA A2 or C3 compared with control arm patients with the same haplotype,[36] as well as overall survival.[37] In patients with resected stage III melanoma, a combination of Melacine for 2 years in combination with low-dose interferon alfa-2b (5 MU/m^2 subcutaneously 3 times per week) was compared with the FDA-approved interferon alfa-2b regimen (20 MU/m^2 by intravenous infusion daily for 5 days over 4 weeks followed by 10 MU/m^2 3 times per week for a total of 52 weeks). Median overall survival was the same (84 months vaccine arm vs 83 months; $P = .56$). Estimated 5-year relapse-free survival was 50% in the vaccine arm versus 40% in the high-dose interferon group.[38] Despite these suggestive data, a further trial of Melacine has not been performed largely due to regulatory, manufacturing, and fiscal concerns.

Donald Morton has been a tireless pioneer in the development of therapeutic cancer vaccines. His early work with BCG suggested nonspecific immune stimulation could mediate antitumor responses. Further trials failed to substantiate the BCG effects; however, in 1984 three melanoma cell lines were used to create Canvaxin. These three lines contained over 20 immunogenic tumor- and melanoma-associated antigens.[39] Cells from these lines were cultured, harvested, washed, and pooled in equal amounts to obtain 25×10^6 viable cells. The combination was then irradiated and frozen in liquid nitrogen. The cells were thawed and administered intradermally every 2 weeks for three to five doses, then monthly for a year. The first two doses were administered along with BCG.

Phase II trials with 157 patients with stage IV melanoma demonstrated a 5-year survival rate of 25% compared with historical controls of 6%.[40,41] Median survival of vaccinated patients was 23 months versus 7.5 months for the historical controls. Additional data suggested that the optimal benefit was seen in patients with resected stage IV disease (5-year overall survival of 33% in vaccinated patients versus 10% in patients who received nonvaccine treatment). In patients with measurable disease, 23% responded (8% complete, 15% partial).[42] Additional statistical work using matched pair analysis further supported the vaccine's effect in patents with resected stage IV disease (5-year overall survival rate 39% in vaccinated patients vs 20% in patients receiving no vaccination, $P = .0009$).[43]

Similar effects were noted in patients with resected stage III melanoma. A phase II trial demonstrated a 49% 5-year overall survival in vaccinated patients versus 37% in historical control patients ($P = .001$).[44]

Based on these results, two multicenter, phase III, randomized trials began in March 1998. The first initially compared Canvaxin plus BCG with interferon alfa-2b in resected stage III patients. The control arm was later changed to placebo plus BCG. The second trial compared Canvaxin plus BCG with placebo plus BCG after complete resection of stage IV melanoma.

By 2005, both trials were halted based on the data safety monitoring committee's assessment that there was little evidence that the vaccine provided significant benefit.[45] No further trails are planned.

Viral Vaccines

Hepatitis B virus (HBV)-associated hepatocellular carcinoma and human papilloma virus (HPV)-associated cervical cancer constitute a substantial segment of the worldwide cancer burden. The introduction of vaccines for these two viral agents has had a dramatic impact on the incidence of these two common malignancies.[46,47]

Persistent HPV infection is associated with the development of cervical cancer. HPV-16 is present in 50% of cervical cancers and high-grade intraepithelial neoplasias. With this as background, Koutsky and colleagues[46] conducted a randomized, double-blind, multicenter trial investigating whether HPV-16 virus-like particle vaccine could reduce the persistence of HPV-16 infection. Two thousand three hundred ninety-two women, ages 16 to 23 years, were randomized to vaccine at day 0, month 2, and month 6 versus placebo. Genital samples were examined before vaccination, 1 month after the final vaccination and every 6 months thereafter. HPV-16 DNA was assessed by polymerase chain reaction. The final analysis included only women who were HPV-16-negative on enrollment. At a median follow-up time of 17.4 months after finishing vaccination, none of the 768 eligible women in the vaccine group had developed HPV-16 infection versus 41 of the 765 women who had received the placebo ($P<.001$). The vaccine had 100% efficacy. All cases of cervical intraepithelial neoplasia occurred in the placebo group. These observations give hope that substantial reductions in the cervical cancer rate may be seen in the near future.

Efforts are underway to use HPV-related vaccines not only for prevention but also for treatment of established disease. In a report by Kenter and colleagues,[48] 15 of 19 vaccinated patients with grade 3 vulvar intraepithelial neoplasia showed responses at 12 months of follow-up with nine having a complete response. These results suggest that reversal of established viral-induced neoplasia is possible.

The systemic use of HBV vaccination in Taiwan has led to remarkable decreases in perinatal hepatitis infections. Babies born to infected mothers who then developed chronic HBV infection dropped from 86%–96% to 12%–14%.[49] After mass vaccination, the incidence of hepatocellular carcinoma in children dropped from 0.70 per 100,000 (1981–1986) to 0.36 (1990–1994; $P<.01$).[50] Because of the substantial infection rate in the general population, general decreases in the hepatocellular carcinoma incidence have yet to be realized; however, these glimpses at what is possible are encouraging.

Unfortunately, the fact that only a few types of cancer appear to be virally mediated, profoundly limits this approach.

ANTIBODY AND ADOPTIVE IMMUNOTHERAPY

Immunotherapy of cancer refers to the area of therapeutics that is based on the manipulation of the immune system to enhance antitumor responses. Although there is considerable overlap, these interventions can arbitrarily be divided into active and passive processes for descriptive purposes. Active immunotherapy refers to strategies that activate host immune effector mechanisms as opposed to passive immunotherapy that involves transfer of humoral or cellular immunity to the host. Immunotherapy can be specific, targeting a specific antigen on a cell, or nonspecific, leading to generalized activation of the immune system. This section focuses primarily on the specific antibody and cell-mediated immune mechanisms that have been exploited for cancer therapy.

Antibody-Mediated Therapy of Cancer—Monoclonal Antibody Therapy

The earliest demonstration of transferring immunity using sera from animals infected with diphtheria to uninfected animals by Behring and Kitsato[51] launched the field of humoral immunotherapy. About the same time, Paul Ehrlich proposed his "side chain hypothesis" alluding to induction of antigen-specific secretion of "preformed receptors" by cells of the immune system; thus conceiving the idea of a "magic bullet."[52] This concept was subsequently deemed to be consistent with generation of an antigen-specific antibody response and—given the limitations in defining these proteins (polyclonal serum)—was used with reasonable success against various infectious diseases. A description of methodology to produce antigen-specific monoclonal antibodies in clinically usable quantity using B cell hybridomas by Kohler and Milstein[53] heralded the dawn of a new era that has opened up numerous potential approaches for immunotherapy, some already with significant success.

Antibody Structure and Function

Immunoglobulins are bifunctional glycoproteins secreted by B lymphocytes in response to appropriate stimuli. Each molecule consists of two heavy chains and two light chains linked by covalent and noncovalent bonds. The amino- or N-terminus of the chains is extremely variable and forms the antigen binding cleft or antigen binding fragment (Fab). The carboxy- or C-terminus of the chains is relatively constant and forms the constant fragment (Fc) portion that interacts with immune effector cells and other components of the immune system including complement (**Fig. 4**). Antibodies are exquisitely antigen specific and constitute a major part of the adaptive immune response, exerting biologic activity by coating the target for destruction by antibody-dependent cell cytotoxicity (ADCC) and complement-mediated cytolysis (CMC).

The earliest monoclonal antibodies used for therapy in humans were produced employing the hybridoma technology and were murine in origin. This posed definite hurdles for use, including generation of human antimouse antibodies and lack of effective interaction with components of the human immune system. Subsequently with advances in genetic engineering, it has become possible to produce chimeric, humanized, and human monoclonal antibodies that exhibit greater efficacy with lesser immunogenicity.

Monoclonal Antibody Therapy for Cancer

Mechanisms of action
Identification of antigens expressed exclusively or preferentially by tumor cells and the ability to make clinically usable amounts of antibodies with defined specificity has made it possible to target these antigens to induce cell death via various mechanisms. These include the following.

Induction of ADCC A number of immune effector cells express Fcγ receptors that can bind to the Fc domain of appropriate antibodies thus providing a bridging mechanism. Recruitment of immune effector cells by monoclonal antibodies bound to tumor cells by their Fab domains results in release of perforin or granzyme molecules and tumor cell death. Clinically this mechanism is believed to play a major role in the antitumor effect exerted by trastuzumab and rituximab (**Fig. 5**).

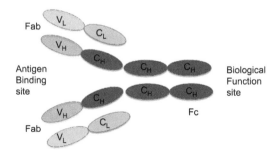

Fig. 4. Antibody structure and function. CH, constant heavy chain; CL, constant light chain; VH, variable heavy chain; VL, variable light chain.

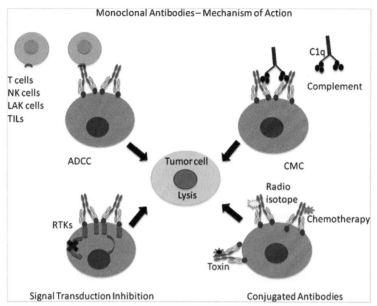

Fig. 5. Monoclonal antibodies mechanism of action. C1q, complement 1q; LAK, lymphokine activated killer cell; NK, natural killer cell; RTK, receptor tyrosine kinase; TIL, tumor infiltrating lymphocyte.

Induction of CMC The complement system comprises a number of soluble proteins that can interact with the Fc domain of antibodies and cause cell lysis. The complement cascade is initiated by binding of the complement 1q (C1q) component to Fc domains of adjoining antibodies bound to the surface of the tumor cell and results in activation of C3 and C4 eventually culminating in formation of the membrane attack complex that disrupts the cell membrane and lysis (see **Fig. 5**).

Inhibition of signal transduction pathways Activation of the receptor tyrosine kinases (RTKs) by an external growth factors results in dimerization of receptors and phosphorylation of the intracellular domain of the RTK leading to cascade activation of signal transduction. Delineation of signal transduction pathways critical for cell growth has made it possible to target them by monoclonal antibodies directed against the extracellular domains of RTKs that prevents dimerization and activation, thus inhibiting cell growth (see **Fig. 5**).

Inhibition of essential adjunct ligands Tumor cells require adjunct mechanisms for continued growth (eg, neoangiogenesis). Identification of critical components involved in angiogenesis (eg, vascular endothelial growth factor [VEGF]) and inhibition by directed monoclonal antibodies have been shown to have clinically relevant benefit against various tumor types. Bevacizumab is now approved for use in colon cancer, RCC, glioblastoma, breast cancer, and lung cancer.

Modulation of cell function Proteins with cell regulatory activity may be expressed on the cell surface and can be targeted by monoclonal antibodies to modulate their function. An excellent example with clinically relevant activity presented recently is that of antibodies directed against the cytotoxic T lymphocyte-associated antigen 4 (CTLA-4) antigen. The CTLA-4 antigen is expressed on the surface of T cells and exerts inhibitory activity interacting with the B7 family of molecules expressed on APCs. Monoclonal antibodies directed against the CTLA-4 protein can block the inhibition normally exerted as a second signal to modulate immune responses after presentation of antigens by APCs. Release from this inhibition results in super activation of the T cell responses, thereby enhancing their antitumor activity. Both ipilimumab and tremelimumab are in development against various tumor types. Antibodies targeting agonist proteins such as CD 137, OX 40, and CD 40 expressed on the cell surface are also in development.

MONOCLONAL ANTIBODY THERAPY OF SOLID TUMORS

This section provides a brief description of the monoclonal antibodies approved by the FDA for various solid tumors, the efficacy data that led to their approval, and major toxicities that need to be kept in mind by the treating physician in the community setting per the most recent approval label (**Table 3**).

Trastuzumab

Trastuzumab (Herceptin) is a humanized IgG1 monoclonal antibody directed against human epidermal growth factor receptor (HER)2. HER2 (or c-erbB2) proto-oncogene encodes for a transmembrane receptor that belongs to the super family of epidermal growth factor receptors. Trastuzumab has been shown, in both in vitro and animal models, to inhibit the proliferation of tumor cells that overexpress HER2 by inhibition of signal transduction. Additionally, trastuzumab can mediate antibody-dependent cell-mediated cytotoxicity (ADCC) and induce tumor cell lysis.

The pivotal trial that compared the benefit of adding trastuzumab to chemotherapy included 469 women with HER 2+ metastatic breast cancer who had not received chemotherapy for metastatic disease. Women who had received adjuvant anthracyclines (n = 188) were randomized to receive paclitaxel or paclitaxel plus trastuzumab while anthracycline-naïve (n = 281) women were randomized to receive adriamycin cyclophosphamide (AC)/epirubicin cyclophosphamide (EC) or AC/EC plus trastuzumab. The addition of trastuzumab to any chemotherapy showed prolonged time to disease progression (7.4 vs 4.6 months), response rate (50% vs 32%), and overall survival (25 vs 20 months). Cardiac dysfunction was most pronounced in the AC plus trastuzumab group, observed in 27% compared with 8% with AC alone, 13% with paclitaxel plus trastuzumab, and 1% with trastuzumab alone. The largest study to evaluate efficacy of trastuzumab as monotherapy in the setting of metastatic breast cancer included 114 women with HER2+ disease who were randomized to 4 mg versus 8 mg induction followed by 2 mg versus 4 mg maintenance. This trial showed an overall response of 35% in women whose tumors expressed 3+ HER2 by immunohistochemistry. In combination with paclitaxel, trastuzumab is approved for treatment of HER2-overexpressing metastatic breast cancer.[54] Trastuzumab is also approved as single agent for treatment of HER2-overexpressing breast cancer in patients who have received one or more chemotherapy regimens for metastatic disease.[55,56]

In the adjuvant setting, a large multinational Herceptin Adjuvant Trial (HERA) compared standard adjuvant chemotherapy with standard adjuvant chemotherapy plus 1 or 2 years of trastuzumab in 5,090 women with nonmetastatic HER2+ breast cancer. An initial report comparing 1,698 controls with 1,703 women who received 1 year of trastuzumab added to their standard chemotherapy; a 36% reduction in the risk of recurrence was noted (DFS 81 vs 74, HR 0.64). The risk of death decreased by 34% (overall survival 92 vs 90, HR 0.66). Trastuzumab is approved as part of

Table 3
Monoclonal antibodies approved for clinical use in humans

Reagent	Approval	Indication
Rituxan (Rituximab)	11/26/1997	Treatment of patients with relapsed or refractory low-grade or follicular, B-cell non-Hodgkin lymphoma
Herceptin (Trastuzumab)	09/25/1998	Treatment of patients with metastatic breast cancer whose tumors overexpress the HER2 protein and who have received 1 or more chemotherapy regimens for their metastatic disease; HER2+ MBC with paclitaxel. Adjuvant therapy of breast cancer
Campath (Alemtuzumab)	05/07/2001	Treatment of patients with B-cell chronic lymphocytic leukemia who have been treated with alkylating agents and who have failed fludarabine therapy
Zevalin (Ibritumomab tiuxetan)	02/19/2002	Treatment of patients with relapsed or refractory low-grade, follicular, or transformed B-cell non-Hodgkin lymphoma, including patients with rituximab (Rituxan) refractory follicular non-Hodgkin lymphoma; the therapeutic regimen includes rituximab, indium-111 ibritumomab tiuxetan, and yttrium-90 ibritumomab tiuxetan
Bexxar (Tositumomab) and (iodine I-131 Tositumomab)	06/27/2003	Treatment of patients with CD20 positive, follicular, non-Hodgkin lymphoma, with and without transformation, whose disease is refractory to rituximab and has relapsed following chemotherapy
Erbitux (Cetuximab)	02/12/2004	Initial treatment of locally or regionally advanced squamous cell carcinoma of the head and neck in combination with radiation therapy. Treatment of patients with recurrent or metastatic squamous cell carcinoma of the head and neck for whom prior platinum-based therapy has failed. Metastatic colorectal cancer
Avastin (Bevacizumab)	02/26/2004	First-line treatment for patients with metastatic colorectal cancer, RCC, breast cancer, non-small cell lung carcinoma, glioblastoma
Vectibix (Panitumumab)	09/27/2006	Treatment of epidermal growth factor receptor (EGFR)-expressing, metastatic colorectal carcinoma with disease progression on or following fluoropyrimidine-, oxaliplatin-, and irinotecan-containing chemotherapy regimens
Arzerra (Ofatumumab)	10/26/2009	Treatment of patients with chronic lymphocytic leukemia refractory to fludarabine and alemtuzumab

Gemtuzumab ozogamicin was approved for treatment of acute myeloid leukemia but has been withdrawn by Pfizer for excessive toxicity (http://www.fda.gov/Safety/MedWatch/Safety Information/SafetyAlertsforHumanMedicalProducts/ucm216458.htm. Accessed March 3, 2011).

a treatment regimen containing doxorubicin, cyclophosphamide, and paclitaxel for the adjuvant treatment of HER2-overexpressing, breast cancer.[57] Trastuzumab is also approved as a single agent, for the adjuvant treatment of HER2-overexpressing node-negative (estrogen receptor [ER]/progesterone receptor [PR] negative or with one high-risk feature) or node-positive breast cancer, following multimodality anthracycline-based therapy.[58]

Cetuximab

Cetuximab (Erbitux) is a chimeric IgG1 monoclonal antibody directed against the epidermal growth factor receptor (EGFR). The EGFR is a member of the family of receptor tyrosine kinases that include EGFR, HER2, HER3, and HER4. Inhibition of signaling by cetuximab can inhibit growth and survival of tumor cells that express EGFR. In addition cetuximab can also mediate ADCC against certain human tumor types in vitro.

The addition of cetuximab to radiation therapy in human tumor xenograft models in mice showed an increase in antitumor effects compared with radiation therapy alone. A phase III study in head and neck cancer showed survival advantage for concomitant cetuximab and radiation compared with radiation alone. Cetuximab is approved in combination with radiation therapy for the initial treatment of locally or regionally advanced squamous cell carcinoma of the head and neck.[59] As a single agent, cetuximab is approved for the treatment of patients with recurrent or metastatic squamous cell carcinoma of the head and neck or who have failed prior platinum-based therapy.[60]

In the setting of colorectal cancer, a phase III study compared treatment with single-agent cetuximab plus best supportive care with best supportive care alone in 572 patients with EGFR-expressing metastatic disease who had previously received fluoropyrimidines, irinotecan, or oxaliplatin, or were not deemed candidates for treatment with these agents. Based on the results of the study, single-agent cetuximab was approved for the treatment of EGFR-expressing metastatic colorectal cancer after failure of both irinotecan- and oxaliplatin-based regimens or intolerance to irinotecan-based regimens. In combination with irinotecan, cetuximab is approved for the treatment of EGFR-expressing metastatic colorectal carcinoma in patients who are refractory to irinotecan-based chemotherapy. Retrospective subset analyses of metastatic or advanced colorectal cancer trials have not shown a treatment benefit for cetuximab in patients whose tumors had Kirsten murine sarcoma virus (K-RAS) mutations in codon 12 or 13. Use of cetuximab is not recommended for the treatment of patients with colorectal cancer who harbor these mutations.[61,62]

Bevacizumab

Bevacizumab (Avastin) is a humanized IgG1 monoclonal antibody directed against the VEGF. The interaction of VEGF with its receptors on the endothelial cells leads to proliferation and new blood vessel formation in in vitro models of angiogenesis. Binding of the monoclonal antibody to VEGF inhibits cell growth and angiogenesis.

Bevacizumab is approved for the first-line or second-line treatment of patients with metastatic carcinoma of the colon or rectum in combination with intravenous 5-fluorouracil–based chemotherapy.[63,64]

Bevacizumab is approved for the first-line treatment of unresectable, locally advanced, recurrent or metastatic nonsquamous non-small cell lung cancer in combination with carboplatin and paclitaxel.[65]

In the setting of breast cancer, a phase III study (ECOG 2100) compared the efficacy of adding bevacizumab to weekly paclitaxel with paclitaxel alone in 722 patients with chemotherapy-naïve metastatic disease. The combination arm showed improvement in progression-free survival (11.8 months vs 5.9 months, HR 0.60) and response rate (36.9% vs 21.2%, $P<.001$) but no difference in overall survival (26.7 months vs 25.2 months, HR 0.88) compared with the control arm. Grade 3–4 hypertension, proteinuria, headache, cerebrovascular ischemia, and infection were more common in the combination arm compared with paclitaxel alone. Bevacizumab was approved for the treatment of patients who have not received chemotherapy for metastatic HER2-negative breast cancer in combination with paclitaxel.[66,67] Bevacizumab is not indicated for patients with breast cancer that has progressed following anthracycline and taxane chemotherapy administered for metastatic disease.

Bevacizumab is approved for the treatment of glioblastoma with progressive disease following prior therapy as a single agent[68] and for the treatment of metastatic RCC in combination with interferon-α.[69,70]

Panitumumab

Panitumumab (Vectibix) is a fully human IgG2 monoclonal antibody directed against EGFR. Signal transduction through the EGFR results in activation of the wild-type K-RAS protein. Cells that harbor activating *K-RAS* mutations, appear independent of EGFR regulation. Panitumumab binds specifically to EGFR and competitively inhibits signaling via EGFR. A retrospective analyses of K-RAS status and outcomes from a phase III study of patients with metastatic colorectal cancer treated with panitumumab showed a significantly better response rate, progression-free survival, and overall survival for patients who harbored the wild-type K-RAS. Use of panitumumab is not recommended for the treatment of colorectal cancer with these mutations.[71] Panitumumab is approved as a single agent for the treatment of EGFR-expressing, metastatic colorectal carcinoma with disease progression on or following fluoropyrimidine-, oxaliplatin-, and irinotecan-containing chemotherapy regimens.[72]

Ipilimumab

Ipilimumab is a fully human IgG1 monoclonal antibody directed against the CTLA-4. The CTLA-4 molecule is expressed on the surface of activated T lymphocytes and acts as an immune checkpoint expressed on the surface of T lymphocytes.[73] Interaction of CTLA-4 with the B7 family of molecules on APCs results in down-regulation of T cell activation. Inhibition of the CTLA-4 molecule results in enhancement of T lymphocyte mediated antitumor activity.[74] Fourteen patients with metastatic melanoma treated with anti-CTLA-4 antibody (MDX-010) in conjunction with HLA-A*0201-restricted peptides from the gp-100 melanoma-associated antigen showed objective cancer regression in three patients (21%; 2 complete and 1 partial responses).[75] This study was later expanded to 56 patients and showed an overall response of 13%; two patients had a complete response (ongoing at 30 and 31 months), and five patients achieved a partial response (durations of 4, 6, 25, 26, and 34 months). Responses were noted to correlate with induction of autoimmunity.[76] Subsequent phase II studies have confirmed clinical activity of this mechanism.[77,78] In a phase III study comparing ipilimumab plus gp-100 vaccine with ipilimumab or the gp-100 vaccine alone in 626 patients with unresectable stage III and stage IV, the disease control rate (CR+PR+SD) was 20.1% for ipilimumab, 28.5% for ipilimumab alone and 11% for gp-100 vaccine alone; there were 14 study drug-related deaths; 7 were associated with immune-related adverse events.[79]

In a community cancer center setting the authors have treated over 100 patients with metastatic melanoma on various phase II, Phase III and expanded access studies since 2005 with less than 1% treatment related mortality (**Fig. 6**).

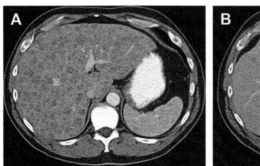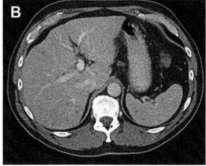

Fig. 6. Pretherapy CT scan (*A*; March 30, 2009) from a patient with advanced metastatic malignant melanoma showing extensive liver metastases. The patient was treated with single agent ipilimumab (10 mg/kg IV every 3 weeks for 4 doses followed by a maintenance dose of 10 mg/kg IV every 3 months). Treatment has been tolerated with no toxicity to date. Posttherapy CT scans (*B*; August 23, 2010) continue to show sustained near-complete response.

CELL-MEDIATED THERAPY OF CANCER—ADOPTIVE CELLULAR THERAPY

Cell-transfer experiments in animals clearly demonstrated that cellular components of the immune system played a key role in rejection of allogeneic grafts and tumors. Based on the previously discussed observations, attempts at adoptive cellular therapy for cancer using normal nonimmunized lymphoid cells began in the 1960s. This area of potential therapeutics underwent a major revival in the 1970s when IL-2 was characterized and shown to be essential and adequate for maintaining lymphocytes in long-term in vitro cultures. Peripheral blood mononuclear cells cultured in IL-2 rich medium were shown to have the ability to lyse natural killer cell insensitive fresh tumor cells in vitro and were described as lymphokine activated killer (LAK) cells.[80] The efficacy of adoptive cell therapy with LAK cells plus IL-2 or immunotherapy with high-dose IL-2 alone in 157 patients with advanced cancer refractory to standard therapy or for whom no standard therapy was available was reported by Rosenberg and colleagues.[81] One hundred and eight patients were treated with LAK cells and IL-2; 49 were treated with high-dose IL-2 alone. Of the 106 evaluable patients treated with LAK cells and IL-2, 8 patients had complete response, 15 had partial responses, and 10 had minor responses. Of the 46 evaluable patients treated with high-dose IL-2 alone, one had a complete response, five had partial responses, and one had a minor response. Subsequent efforts led to the isolation, enrichment, and use of lymphocytes obtained from fresh autologous tumors as a source of effector cells.[82] In a pilot study, 12 patients (6 melanoma, 4 RCC, 1 breast cancer, and 1 colon cancer) were treated with tumor infiltrating lymphocytes (TILs) and IL-2. One patient with melanoma, one with RCC, and one patient with breast cancer experienced partial responses.[83] Despite an impressive increase in the percentage of patients responding to these cellular therapies, the complete and durable response rate was similar to high-dose IL2 alone. Dudley and colleagues[84] reported the cumulative experience from three adoptive TIL therapy studies employing nonmyeloablative (NMA) lymphodepletion (preparative chemotherapy consisting of fludarabine and cyclophosphamide), NMA with 2 Gy total body irradiation (TBI), or NMA with 12 Gy TBI in 93 patients with metastatic melanoma. The overall response was 49% with NMA, 52% with NMA plus 2 Gy, and 72% with NMA plus 12 Gy. There was one treatment-related death. While results of the LAK cell and TIL adoptive therapy are impressive and provocative, the intensity of labor and need for basic and laboratory support involved precludes them to be considered as standard therapeutic modalities in a community cancer center at present time.[84]

ACKNOWLEDGMENTS

The authors thank Cissy Swartz for her assistance in the preparation of this manuscript.

REFERENCES

1. Richardson MA, Ramirez T, Russell NC, et al. Coley toxins immunotherapy: a retrospective review. Altern Ther Health Med 1999;5:42–7.
2. Rosenberg SA, Mule JJ, Spiess PJ, et al. Regression of established pulmonary metastases and subcutaneous tumor mediated by the systemic administration of high-dose recombinant interleukin 2. J Exp Med 1985;161:1169–88.
3. Rosenberg SA, Lotze MT, Muul LM, et al. Observations on the systemic administration of autologous lymphokine-activated killer cells and recombinant interleukin-2 to patients with metastatic cancer. N Engl J Med 1985;313:1485–92.
4. Morgan DA, Ruscetti FW, Gallo R. Selective in vitro growth of T lymphocytes from normal human bone marrows. Science 1976;193:1007–8.
5. Gemlo BT, Palladino MA Jr, Jaffe HS, et al. Circulating cytokines in patients with metastatic cancer treated with recombinant interleukin 2 and lymphokine-activated killer cells. Cancer Res 1988;48:5864–7.
6. Wood TF, DiFronzo LA, Rose DM, et al. Does complete resection of melanoma metastatic to solid intra-abdominal organs improve survival? Ann Surg Oncol 2001;8:658–62.
7. Atkins MB, Lotze MT, Dutcher JP, et al. High-dose recombinant interleukin 2 therapy for patients with metastatic melanoma: analysis of 270 patients treated between 1985 and 1993. J Clin Oncol 1999;17:2105–16.
8. Kammula US, White DE, Rosenberg SA. Trends in the safety of high dose bolus interleukin-2 administration in patients with metastatic cancer. Cancer 1998;83: 797–805.
9. Fyfe G, Fisher RI, Rosenberg SA, et al. Results of treatment of 255 patients with metastatic renal cell carcinoma who received high-dose recombinant interleukin-2 therapy. J Clin Oncol 1995;13:688–96.
10. McDermott DF, Regan MM, Clark JI, et al. Randomized phase III trial of high-dose interleukin-2 versus subcutaneous interleukin-2 and interferon in patients with metastatic renal cell carcinoma. J Clin Oncol 2005;23:133–41.
11. Klapper JA, Downey SG, Smith FO, et al. High-dose interleukin-2 for the treatment of metastatic renal cell carcinoma: a retrospective analysis of response and survival in patients treated in the surgery branch at the National Cancer Institute between 1986 and 2006. Cancer 2008;113:293–301.
12. Yang JC, Sherry RM, Steinberg SM, et al. Randomized study of high-dose and low-dose interleukin-2 in patients with metastatic renal cancer. J Clin Oncol 2003;21:3127–32.
13. Available at: http://www.proleukin.com/health-care-professional/index.jsp. Accessed September 18, 2010.
14. Parkhurst MR, Salgaller ML, Southwood S, et al. Improved induction of melanoma-reactive CTL with peptides from the melanoma antigen gp100 modified at HLA-A*0201-binding residues. J Immunol 1996;157:2539–48.

15. Rosenberg SA, Yang JC, Schwartzentruber DJ, et al. Immunologic and therapeutic evaluation of a synthetic peptide vaccine for the treatment of patients with metastatic melanoma. Nat Med 1998;4:321–7.
16. Sosman JA, Carrillo C, Urba WJ, et al. Three phase II cytokine working group trials of gp100 (210M) peptide plus high-dose interleukin-2 in patients with HLA-A2-positive advanced melanoma. J Clin Oncol 2008;26:2292–8.
17. Schwartzentruber DJ, Lawson D, Richards J, et al. A phase III multi-institutional randomized study of immunization with the gp100: 209–217(210M) peC followed by high-dose IL-2 compared with high-dose IL-2 alone in patients with metastatic melanoma. J Clin Oncol 2009;27:CRA9001 [meeting abstracts].
18. Kirkwood JM, Ernstoff MS. Interferons in the treatment of human cancer. J Clin Oncol 1984;2:336–52.
19. Kirkwood JM, Strawderman MH, Ernstoff MS, et al. Interferon alfa-2b adjuvant therapy of high-risk resected cutaneous melanoma: the Eastern Cooperative Oncology Group Trial EST 1684. J Clin Oncol 1996;14:7–17.
20. Kirkwood JM, Ibrahim JG, Sondak VK, et al. High- and low-dose interferon alfa-2b in high-risk melanoma: first analysis of intergroup trial E1690/S9111/C9190. J Clin Oncol 2000;18:2444–58.
21. Kirkwood JM, Ibrahim JG, Sosman JA, et al. High-dose interferon alfa-2b significantly prolongs relapse-free and overall survival compared with the GM2-KLH/QS-21 vaccine in patients with resected stage IIB-III melanoma: results of intergroup trial E1694/S9512/C509801. J Clin Oncol 2001;19:2370–80.
22. Mocellin S, Pasquali S, Rossi CR, et al. Interferon alpha adjuvant therapy in patients with high-risk melanoma: a systematic review and meta-analysis. J Natl Cancer Inst 2010;102:493–501.
23. Eggermont AM, Suciu S, Santinami M, et al. Adjuvant therapy with pegylated interferon alfa-2b versus observation alone in resected stage III melanoma: final results of EORTC 18991, a randomised phase III trial. Lancet 2008;372:117–26.
24. Rosenberg SA, Yang JC, Restifo NP. Cancer immunotherapy: moving beyond current vaccines. Nat Med 2004;10:909–15.
25. Disis ML, Bernhard H, Shiota FM, et al. Granulocyte-macrophage colony-stimulating factor: an effective adjuvant for protein and peptide-based vaccines. Blood 1996;88:202–10.
26. Overwijk WW, de Visser KE, Tirion FH, et al. Immunological and antitumor effects of IL-23 as a cancer vaccine adjuvant. J Immunol 2006;176:5213–22.
27. Kantoff PW, Higano CS, Shore ND, et al. Sipuleucel-T immunotherapy for castration-resistant prostate cancer. N Engl J Med 2010;363:411–22.
28. Kantoff PW, Schuetz TJ, Blumenstein BA, et al. Overall survival analysis of a phase II randomized controlled trial of a Poxviral-based PSA-targeted immunotherapy in metastatic castration-resistant prostate cancer. J Clin Oncol 2010;28:1099–105.
29. Bedikian AY, Richards J, Kharkevitch D, et al. A phase 2 study of high-dose Allovectin-7 in patients with advanced metastatic melanoma. Melanoma Res 2010; 20:218–26.
30. Bedikian AY, Del Vecchio M. Allovectin-7 therapy in metastatic melanoma. Expert Opin Biol Ther 2008;8:839–44.
31. Berd D, Maguire HC Jr, Schuchter LM, et al. Autologous hapten-modified melanoma vaccine as postsurgical adjuvant treatment after resection of nodal metastases. J Clin Oncol 1997;15:2359–70.
32. Berd D, Sato T, Maguire HC Jr, et al. Immunopharmacologic analysis of an autologous, hapten-modified human melanoma vaccine. J Clin Oncol 2004;22:403–15.

33. Available at: http://www.clinicaltrials.gov/ct2/show/NCT00477906?term= NCT00477906&rank=1. Accessed September 27, 2010.

34. Mitchell MS, Kan-Mitchell J, Kempf RA, et al. Active specific immunotherapy for melanoma: phase I trial of allogeneic lysates and a novel adjuvant. Cancer Res 1988;48:5883–93.

35. Sondak VK, Liu PY, Tuthill RJ, et al. Adjuvant immunotherapy of resected, intermediate-thickness, node-negative melanoma with an allogeneic tumor vaccine: overall results of a randomized trial of the Southwest Oncology Group. J Clin Oncol 2002;20:2058–66.

36. Sosman JA, Unger JM, Liu PY, et al. Adjuvant immunotherapy of resected, intermediate-thickness, node-negative melanoma with an allogeneic tumor vaccine: impact of HLA class I antigen expression on outcome. J Clin Oncol 2002;20:2067–75.

37. Sondak VK, Sosman J, Unger J. Significant impact of HLA class I allele expression on outcome in melanoma patients treated with an allogeneic melanoma cell lysate vaccine: final analysis of SWOG-9035 [abstract]. J Clin Oncol 2004;22: 710s.

38. Mitchell MS, Abrams J, Thompson JA, et al. Randomized trial of an allogeneic melanoma lysate vaccine with low-dose interferon Alfa-2b compared with high-dose interferon Alfa-2b for Resected stage III cutaneous melanoma. J Clin Oncol 2007;25:2078–85.

39. Kadison AS, Morton DL. Immunotherapy of malignant melanoma. Surg Clin North Am 2003;83:343–70.

40. Morton DL, Barth A. Vaccine therapy for malignant melanoma. CA Cancer J Clin 1996;46:225–44.

41. Morton DL, Nizze A, Hoon D. Improved survival of advanced stage IV melanoma following active immunotherapy: correlation with immune response to melanoma vaccine. Proc Am Soc Clin Oncol 1993;12:391.

42. Morton DL, Foshag LJ, Hoon DS, et al. Prolongation of survival in metastatic melanoma after active specific immunotherapy with a new polyvalent melanoma vaccine. Ann Surg 1992;216:463–82.

43. Hsueh EC, Essner R, Foshag LJ, et al. Prolonged survival after complete resection of disseminated melanoma and active immunotherapy with a therapeutic cancer vaccine. J Clin Oncol 2002;20:4549–54.

44. Morton DL, Hsueh EC, Essner R, et al. Prolonged survival of patients receiving active immunotherapy with Canvaxin therapeutic polyvalent vaccine after complete resection of melanoma metastatic to regional lymph nodes. Ann Surg 2002;236:438–48 [discussion: 48–9].

45. Morton DL, Mozzillo N, Thompson JF, et al. An international, randomized, phase III trial of bacillus Calmette-Guerin (BCG) plus allogeneic melanoma vaccine (MCV) or placebo after complete resection of melanoma metastatic to regional or distant sites. Paper presented at: American Society of Clinical Oncology Annual Meeting Part 1; 2007. J Clin Oncol 2007;25(Suppl 20):18S.

46. Koutsky LA, Ault KA, Wheeler CM, et al. A controlled trial of a human papillomavirus type 16 vaccine. N Engl J Med 2002;347:1645–51.

47. Sun Z, Zhu Y, Stjernsward J, et al. Design and compliance of HBV vaccination trial on newborns to prevent hepatocellular carcinoma and 5-year results of its pilot study. Cancer Detect Prev 1991;15:313–8.

48. Kenter GG, Welters MJ, Valentijn AR, et al. Vaccination against HPV-16 oncoproteins for vulvar intraepithelial neoplasia. N Engl J Med 2009;361:1838–47.

49. Hsu HM, Lu CF, Lee SC, et al. Seroepidemiologic survey for hepatitis B virus infection in Taiwan: the effect of hepatitis B mass immunization. J Infect Dis 1999;179:367–70.

50. Chang MH, Chen CJ, Lai MS, et al. Universal hepatitis B vaccination in Taiwan and the incidence of hepatocellular carcinoma in children. Taiwan Childhood Hepatoma Study Group. N Engl J Med 1997;336:1855–9.

51. Behring E, Kitasato S. Ueber das Zustandekommen der Diphtherie-Immunitat und der Tetanus-Immunitat bei thieren. Deutsche medizinsche Wochenschrift 1890;16:1113–4. In: Milestones in microbiology: 1556 to 1940 [translated and edited by Thomas D. Brock]. ASM Press; 1998. p. 138.

52. Ehrlich P. The relationship existing between constitution, distribution and pharmacological action. In: Himmelweite F, Marquardt M, Dale H, editors. The collected papers of Paul Ehrlich, vol. 1. London, New York: Pergamon Press; 1956. p. 596–618.

53. Kohler G, Milstein C. Continuous cultures of fused cells secreting antibody of predefined specificity. Nature 1975;256:495–7.

54. Slamon DJ, Leyland-Jones B, Shak S, et al. Use of chemotherapy plus a monoclonal antibody against HER2 for metastatic breast cancer that overexpresses HER2. N Engl J Med 2001;344:783–92.

55. Cobleigh MA, Vogel CL, Tripathy D, et al. Multinational study of the efficacy and safety of humanized anti-HER2 monoclonal antibody in women who have HER2-overexpressing metastatic breast cancer that has progressed after chemotherapy for metastatic disease. J Clin Oncol 1999;17:2639–48.

56. Vogel CL, Cobleigh MA, Tripathy D, et al. Efficacy and safety of trastuzumab as a single agent in first-line treatment of HER2-overexpressing metastatic breast cancer. J Clin Oncol 2002;20:719–26.

57. Romond EH, Perez EA, Bryant J, et al. Trastuzumab plus adjuvant chemotherapy for operable HER2-positive breast cancer. N Engl J Med 2005;353:1673–84.

58. Piccart-Gebhart MJ, Procter M, Leyland-Jones B, et al. Trastuzumab after adjuvant chemotherapy in HER2-positive breast cancer. N Engl J Med 2005;353:1659–72.

59. Bonner JA, Harari PM, Giralt J, et al. Radiotherapy plus cetuximab for squamous-cell carcinoma of the head and neck. N Engl J Med 2006;354:567–78.

60. Vermorken JB, Trigo J, Hitt R, et al. Open-label, uncontrolled, multicenter phase II study to evaluate the efficacy and toxicity of cetuximab as a single agent in patients with recurrent and/or metastatic squamous cell carcinoma of the head and neck who failed to respond to platinum-based therapy. J Clin Oncol 2007; 25:2171–7.

61. Sobrero AF, Maurel J, Fehrenbacher L, et al. EPIC: phase III trial of cetuximab plus irinotecan after fluoropyrimidine and oxaliplatin failure in patients with metastatic colorectal cancer. J Clin Oncol 2008;26:2311–9.

62. Jonker DJ, O'Callaghan CJ, Karapetis CS, et al. Cetuximab for the treatment of colorectal cancer. N Engl J Med 2007;357:2040–8.

63. Hurwitz H, Fehrenbacher L, Novotny W, et al. Bevacizumab plus irinotecan, fluorouracil, and leucovorin for metastatic colorectal cancer. N Engl J Med 2004;350: 2335–42.

64. Giantonio BJ, Catalano PJ, Meropol NJ, et al. Bevacizumab in combination with oxaliplatin, fluorouracil, and leucovorin (FOLFOX4) for previously treated metastatic colorectal cancer: results from the Eastern Cooperative Oncology Group Study E3200. J Clin Oncol 2007;25:1539–44.

65. Sandler A, Gray R, Perry MC, et al. Paclitaxel-carboplatin alone or with bevacizumab for non-small-cell lung cancer. N Engl J Med 2006;355:2542–50.

66. Miller K, Wang M, Gralow J, et al. Paclitaxel plus bevacizumab versus paclitaxel alone for metastatic breast cancer. N Engl J Med 2007;357:2666–76.
67. Robert NJ, Dieras V, Glaspy J, et al. RIBBON-1: Randomized double-blind placebo-controlled, phase III trial of chemotherapy with or without bevacizumab (B) for first-line treatment of HER2-negative locally recurrent or metastatic breast cancer (MBC). Paper presented at: American Society of Clinical Oncology, 2009. Orlando (FL). J Clin Oncol 2009;27(Suppl 15):A1005.
68. Friedman HS, Prados MD, Wen PY, et al. Bevacizumab alone and in combination with irinotecan in recurrent glioblastoma. J Clin Oncol 2009;27:4733–40.
69. Escudier B, Bellmunt J, Negrier S, et al. Final results of the phase III, randomized, double-blind AVOREN trial of first-line devacizumab (BEV) + interferon-alpha2a (IFN) in metastatic renal cell carcinoma (mRCC). Paper presented at: American Society of Clinical Oncology, 2009. Orlando (FL). J Clin Oncol 2009;27(Suppl 15): A5020.
70. Escudier B, Bellmunt J, Negrier S, et al. Phase III trial of bevacizumab plus interferon alfa-2a in patients with metastatic renal cell carcinoma (AVOREN): final analysis of overall survival. J Clin Oncol 2010;28:2144–50.
71. Amado RG, Wolf M, Peeters M, et al. Wild-type KRAS is required for panitumumab efficacy in patients with metastatic colorectal cancer. J Clin Oncol 2008; 26:1626–34.
72. Van Cutsem E, Peeters M, Siena S, et al. Open-label phase III trial of panitumumab plus best supportive care compared with best supportive care alone in patients with chemotherapy-refractory metastatic colorectal cancer. J Clin Oncol 2007;25:1658–64.
73. Lindsten T, Lee KP, Harris ES, et al. Characterization of CTLA-4 structure and expression on human T cells. J Immunol 1993;151:3489–99.
74. Leach DR, Krummel MF, Allison JP. Enhancement of antitumor immunity by CTLA-4 blockade. Science 1996;271:1734–6.
75. Phan GQ, Yang JC, Sherry RM, et al. Cancer regression and autoimmunity induced by cytotoxic T lymphocyte-associated antigen 4 blockade in patients with metastatic melanoma. Proc Natl Acad Sci U S A 2003;100:8372–7.
76. Attia P, Phan GQ, Maker AV, et al. Autoimmunity correlates with tumor regression in patients with metastatic melanoma treated with anti-cytotoxic T-lymphocyte antigen-4. J Clin Oncol 2005;23:6043–53.
77. Weber J, Thompson JA, Hamid O, et al. A randomized, double-blind, placebo-controlled, phase II study comparing the tolerability and efficacy of ipilimumab administered with or without prophylactic budesonide in patients with unresectable stage III or IV melanoma. Clin Cancer Res 2009;15:5591–8.
78. O'Day SJ, Maio M, Chiarion-Sileni V, et al. Efficacy and safety of ipilimumab monotherapy in patients with pretreated advanced melanoma: a multicenter single-arm phase II study. Ann Oncol 2010;21:1712–7.
79. Hodi FS, O'Day SJ, McDermott DF, et al. Improved survival with Ipilimumab in patients with metastatic melanoma. N Engl J Med 2010;363:711–23.
80. Grimm EA, Mazumder A, Zhang HZ, et al. Lymphokine-activated killer cell phenomenon. Lysis of natural killer-resistant fresh solid tumor cells by interleukin 2-activated autologous human peripheral blood lymphocytes. J Exp Med 1982; 155:1823–41.
81. Rosenberg SA, Lotze MT, Muul LM, et al. A progress report on the treatment of 157 patients with advanced cancer using lymphokine-activated killer cells and interleukin-2 or high-dose interleukin-2 alone. N Engl J Med 1987;316: 889–97.

82. Rosenberg SA, Spiess P, Lafreniere R. A new approach to the adoptive immuno-therapy of cancer with tumor-infiltrating lymphocytes. Science 1986;233: 1318–21.

83. Topalian SL, Solomon D, Avis FP, et al. Immunotherapy of patients with advanced cancer using tumor-infiltrating lymphocytes and recombinant interleukin-2: a pilot study. J Clin Oncol 1988;6:839–53.

84. Dudley ME, Yang JC, Sherry R, et al. Adoptive cell therapy for patients with meta-static melanoma: evaluation of intensive myeloablative chemoradiation prepara-tive regimens. J Clin Oncol 2008;26:5233–9.

Breast Cancer Care in the Community: Challenges, Opportunities, and Outcomes

Diana Dickson-Witmer, MD[a,b,*], Aaron D. Bleznak, MD[c,d],
John S. Kennedy, MD[e], Andrew K. Stewart, MA[f],
Bryan E. Palis, MA[f], Lisa Bailey, MD[g], Alison L. Laidley, MD, FRCS(C)[h],
Emily J. Penman, MD[a,b]

KEYWORDS

- Community cancer center • Breast surgeon volume
- NQF measures • Mastery of Breast Surgery Program
- Quality of cancer care • Breast cancer • Outcomes

According to the World Health Organization, breast cancer comprises 22.8% of all cancers in women worldwide.[1] In the United States, 80% of patients with breast cancer are treated by community breast surgeons. This article discusses the challenges community breast surgeons face and some of the ways that the quality of care delivered could be monitored and improved.

An increasing body of literature suggests that there are, between hospitals of different sizes and resources, disparities in outcomes of cancer care. Our examination of the problem of disparities in breast cancer outcomes is framed by the Donabedian paradigm of the 3 domains of quality assessment: structure, process, and outcomes.[2]

[a] Department of Surgery, Christiana Care Breast Center, Helen F Graham Cancer Center, 4701 Ogletown-Stanton Road, Newark, DE 19713, USA
[b] Thomas Jefferson Medical College, 1025 Walnut Street, Philadelphia, PA 19107, USA
[c] Department of Surgery, Lehigh Valley Health Network, John and Dorothy Morgan Cancer Center, 1240 South Cedar Crest Boulevard Suite 210, Allentown, PA 18103, USA
[d] University of South Florida School of Medicine, Tampa, FL 33612, USA
[e] DeKalb Medical Center, 2665 North Decatur Road, Suite 730, Decatur, GA 30033, USA
[f] American College of Surgeons, Commission on Cancer, National Cancer Data Base, 633 North Saint Clair Street, Chicago, IL 60611, USA
[g] Bay Area Breast Surgeons, Inc, 3300 Webster Street, Suite 212, Oakland, CA 94609, USA
[h] Texas Breast Specialists, 7777 Forest Lane #C614, Dallas, TX 75230, USA
* Corresponding author. Department of Surgery, Christiana Care Breast Center, Helen F Graham Cancer Center, 4701 Ogletown-Stanton Road, Newark, DE 19713.
E-mail address: DDickson-Witmer@Christianacare.org

Surg Oncol Clin N Am 20 (2011) 555–580
doi:10.1016/j.soc.2011.01.007
1055-3207/11/$ – see front matter © 2011 Elsevier Inc. All rights reserved.

surgonc.theclinics.com

The goal of all our quality improvement efforts as health care providers is to improve the outcomes for communities and patients.

Drs Bleznak and Kennedy and Mr Stewart and Mr Palis begin this article with an analysis of clinical process and outcomes data from the Commission on Cancer (CoC). They compare and contrast performance among hospitals in different categories of CoC accreditation. The hospitals in the CoC program treat 70% of patients newly diagnosed with cancer in the United States. Also, in the domain of outcomes assessment, Dr Bailey reviews the performance of breast surgeons according to the volume of patients with breast cancer treated. She presents evidence supporting the premise that breast-focused, high-volume breast surgeons achieve better outcomes for their patients.

In the domain of process, Dr Laidley describes the ways the American Society of Breast Surgeons is working to improve the quality of breast cancer care in the United States through its Mastery of Breast Surgery Program. In the domain of structure, Drs Penman and Dickson-Witmer relate the way a community cancer center has worked collaboratively with a mix of hospital-based, employed, and private practice physicians to develop a multidisciplinary breast program with continuous processes of quality improvement. In a separate article of this issue, Dr Winchester describes the ways that all 3 domains of quality are addressed by the National Accreditation Program for Breast Centers with the goal of improving breast cancer care across a broad spectrum of delivery environments.

AN ANALYSIS OF PERFORMANCE AMONG CANCER PROGRAMS IN DIFFERENT CATEGORIES OF COC ACCREDITATION
The Mission of the CoC

The CoC, established in 1922 by the American College of Surgeons, is a consortium of more than 100 individuals representing more than 50 national professional organizations. The commission's efforts are designed to improve the quality of cancer care in all categories of cancer programs, so that patients may receive the highest quality of care, with the greatest possible probability of cure, without leaving their local commission-accredited cancer program (of which there are >1500 in the United States).

The commission improves the quality of cancer care by establishing standards for multidisciplinary care, outreach efforts, quality of cancer data collected, and use of information about each institution's treatments and outcomes as measured against nationally recognized benchmarks. Just more than 70% of patients newly diagnosed with cancer in the United States receive all or part of their care in a CoC-accredited program each year. The commission accredits more than 1500 cancer programs in the United States, surveying each program every 3 years to evaluate compliance with 36 standards. Patient-level data from accredited programs are reported to the National Cancer Data Base (NCDB) of the CoC following nationally standardized data collection processes and transmission protocols. These data are compiled in the largest cancer database in the world, housing information on demographics, disease site, stage, treatment, and survival for more than 26 million patients. The NCDB, a joint program of the American College of Surgeons' CoC and the American Cancer Society, is the data source used in this article for the examination of similarities and differences between cancer programs of different types regarding surgical treatment of women with breast cancer, performance on the CoC's breast-related quality-of-care indicators, and survival of patients with breast cancer.

For purposes of this article, patients with breast cancer in the NCDB were identified by the topography code C50.X according to the International Classification of Disease-Oncology third edition. Hospital cancer registries abstracted cases with the Facility Oncology Registry Data Standards manuals, a standardized set of data elements and definitions, using information provided by both patients and hospital medical information systems.

Patient-level data were selected from the NCDB in 2 cohorts based on the time of diagnosis. There were 319,080 patients with breast cancer registered in the NCDB between January 1, 2007, and December 31, 2008. The second cohort comprised 271,328 patients with 5-year follow-up diagnosed between January 1, 2002, and December 31, 2003. For analysis, both patient cohorts were limited to adult female patients older than 18 years diagnosed with either 1 malignant or the first of 2 or more malignant primaries. Aggregate-level hospital data were obtained from the Cancer Program Practice Profile Reports (CP3R), a program of the NCDB, from 1397 participating accredited facilities.

Descriptive statistics were calculated for all variables presented in the analysis. Categorical variables were assessed for significance using the 2-sided z tests of proportional difference. Five-year overall survival rates were calculated from the date of diagnosis to death or the last follow-up. Patients diagnosed from 2002 to 2003 were evaluated for survival outcome and had a minimum of 5 years of follow-up data. Survival was estimated by the relative survival method, calculated as a ratio of observed survival over expected survival of the general US population. Cox proportional hazards model was used to determine the risk of mortality on age, insurance status, race/ethnicity, ZIP code–level income, tumor grade, the Charleson-Deyo comorbidity index, hospital type, and treatment. Hazard ratios with 95% confidence intervals were generated; hazard ratio greater than 1.0 indicates an increased likelihood of death. The level of statistical significance was set at $P<.05$. All analyses were generated using SPSS 17.0.1 (SPSS, Inc, Chicago, IL, USA).

Table 1 displays some of the criteria for CoC program category designation. Seventy-two percent of programs are in 1 of the 2 community hospital categories, and just more than 20% of programs are Teaching Hospital Cancer Programs, Network Cancer Programs, or National Cancer Institute (NCI)-designated Comprehensive Cancer Programs. **Fig. 1** displays the average annual breast cancer case volume by CoC accreditation category (for diagnosis years 2005–2007). Cancer programs have been divided into 4 groups based on quartile break points. Note that 86% of community hospital cancer programs have fewer than 106 analytical breast cancer cases annually, whereas 86% of NCI comprehensive cancer centers have more than 106 analytical breast cancer cases annually.

Despite the large differences in case volume and in-house resource availability shown in **Table 1**, the CoC holds community and comprehensive community cancer programs to the same set of high standards to which it holds academic and NCI centers. These CoC standards, revised every 5 to 6 years, address not only treatment planning multidisciplinary tumor boards, and data standards, but also adherence to nationally recognized treatment standards, use of College of American Pathologists' reporting guidelines, quality improvement activities, and certification of radiation oncology facilities. There are differences in breast cancer case volume and in research and oncology subspecialty availability between CoC program categories. Two of these variables, volume and subspecialty expertise, have been suggested as factors contributing to outcomes variations for several malignancies and at times have been used as justification for recommendations for centralization of cancer care.[3,4]

Demographics

The reported comorbidities, an assessment of patients' overall medical status as measured by the Charleson-Deyo method, and American Joint Committee on Cancer (AJCC) stage of breast cancer (**Fig. 2**) did not vary across categories, but the age distribution of the women varies by program category. Younger women are more likely

Table 1
CoC program category designation (abstracted from the CoC Cancer Program Standards 2009 Revised Edition)

CoC Program Category	Annual Newly Diagnosed Cancer Cases	Clinical Research	Residencies and Medical School Affiliation	Diagnostic and Treatment Services	Oncology Specialties
Community Hospital Cancer Program	100–649	Optional	Optional	Available but referral common for a portion of treatment	Medical staff is board certified in the major medical specialties
Community Hospital Comprehensive Cancer Program	≥650	Required	Optional	Available on site or by referral	Medical staff is board certified in the major medical specialties
Teaching Hospital Cancer Program	No requirement	Required	≥4 including medical and surgical required	Available on site or by referral	Medical staff is board certified in the major medical specialties including oncology
Network Cancer Program	No requirement	Required	Optional	Available within network	Medical staff is board certified in the major medical specialties including oncology
NCI-designated Comprehensive Cancer Center Program	No requirement	Required; basic science research required	Optional	Available on site	Medical staff is board certified in the major medical specialties including oncology

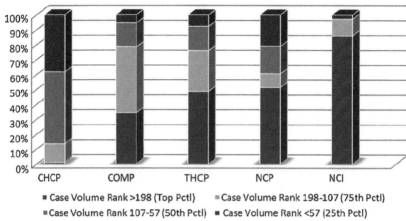

Fig. 1. Facility category by average annual breast cancer case volume. CHCP, Community Hospital Cancer Program; COMP, Community Hospital Comprehensive Cancer Program; NCP, Network Cancer Program; THCP, Teaching Hospital Cancer Program.

to present to NCI-designated, network, and teaching hospital programs (**Fig. 3**). More than 45% of all women diagnosed between 18 and 49 years of age were treated at the 346 networked, academic, or research centers. At the NCI-designated programs, one third of patients treated for breast cancer were younger than 50 years, in contrast to 21.4% at community programs and 23.3% at comprehensive community programs.

National Quality Forum quality measures
Since 2005, the CoC has been using NCDB data to report back to programs on their performance against National Quality Forum (NQF)-endorsed quality of cancer care measures. Three of these measures relate to breast cancer care:

1. Radiation therapy is administered within 1 year (365 days) of diagnosis for women younger than 70 years receiving breast-conserving surgery for breast cancer.

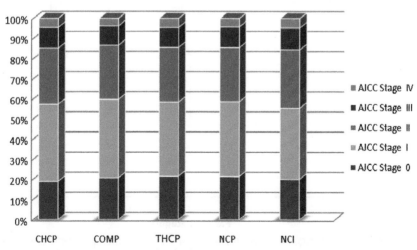

Fig. 2. Derived AJCC stage group by facility category, 2007 to 2008 (N = 318,708). CHCP, Community Hospital Cancer Program; COMP, Community Hospital Comprehensive Cancer Program; NCP, Network Cancer Program; THCP, Teaching Hospital Cancer Program.

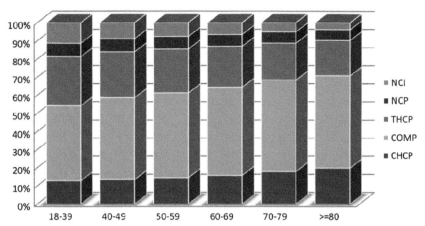

Fig. 3. Facility category by age at diagnosis, 2007 to 2008 (N = 326,896). CHCP, Community Hospital Cancer Program; COMP, Community Hospital Comprehensive Cancer Program; NCP, Network Cancer Program; THCP, Teaching Hospital Cancer Program.

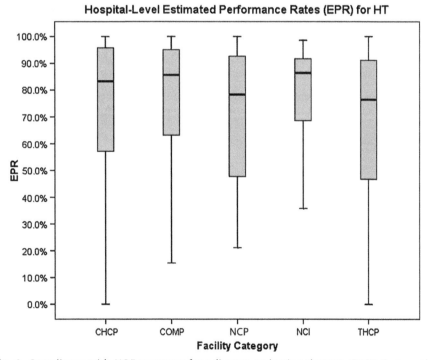

Fig. 4. Compliance with NQF measures for adjuvant endocrine therapy. CHCP, Community Hospital Cancer Program; COMP, Community Hospital Comprehensive Cancer Program; HT, hormonal therapy; NCP, Network Cancer Program; THCP, Teaching Hospital Cancer Program.

2. Tamoxifen or third-generation aromatase inhibitor is considered or administered within 1 year (365 days) of diagnosis for women with AJCC T1c N0 M0 or stage II or III hormone receptor–positive breast cancer.
3. Combination chemotherapy is considered or administered within 4 months (120 days) of diagnosis for women younger than 70 years with AJCC T1c N0 M0 or stage II or III hormone receptor–negative breast cancer.

Two of the CoC's quality of breast care measures assess the appropriate use of systemic therapies. Performance on these indicators (**Figs. 4** and **5**) is equal across the 5 categories of CoC-accredited programs; no significant differences are noted. Adjuvant hormonal therapy, either tamoxifen or an aromatase inhibitor, is reported as being prescribed for between 66.9% and 78.6% of women younger than 70 years with estrogen receptor (ER)–positive, AJCC stage I (T1c), stage II, and stage III breast cancers. Multiagent chemotherapy is administered or recommended to between 81.4% and 86% of eligible women.

The final NQF-endorsed breast cancer measure deployed by the CoC assesses the use of adjuvant radiation therapy for women younger than 70 years who undergo breast-conserving surgery (**Fig. 6**) and is also met without statistically significant differences across CoC categories, with performance rates ranging from 81.2% to 88.4%.

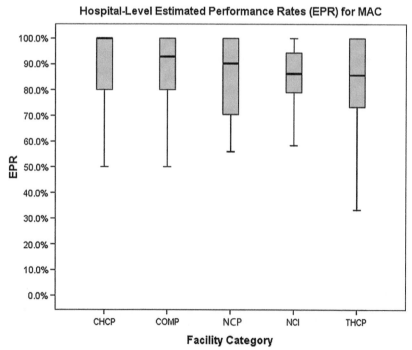

Fig. 5. Compliance with NQF measure for adjuvant chemotherapy. CHCP, Community Hospital Cancer Program; COMP, Community Hospital Comprehensive Cancer Program; MAC, multiagent chemotherapy; NCP, Network Cancer Program; THCP, Teaching Hospital Cancer Program.

These 3 breast NQF measures are currently available to all CoC-accredited hospitals in the form of CP3R, using data that are approximately 18 months old. A new initiative of the CoC, currently being beta tested across the country at 65 facilities, is the Rapid Quality Reporting System (RQRS). This effort, which requires timely abstracting of selected data elements, provides institutions with almost real-time quality metrics on their patients with breast cancer using the same 3 NQF measures. The goal of this initiative was to enhance the ability for cancer programs to identify quality issues and rectify them in a timely fashion, preventing patients from "falling through the cracks."

Surgical Treatment Administered

Overall rates of breast-conserving surgery were 74.3%, 73.6%, 51.5%, and 23.6% for stages 0, I, II, and III, respectively. **Table 2** shows that there was some observed variation among the categories of cancer programs, with Community Hospital Cancer Programs reporting the highest breast conservation rates for stages 0, I, and II at 77.6%, 75%, and 52.6%, respectively. The NCI programs had, on average, significantly lower rates of breast-conserving surgery for stages 0 and I (69.1% and 70.3%, respectively), which might be explained by the larger proportion of younger women seen at the institutions of NCI. A program with a higher percentage of very young women would also be expected to have a higher percentage of mutation carriers, for whom bilateral total mastectomy is often the most appropriate procedure

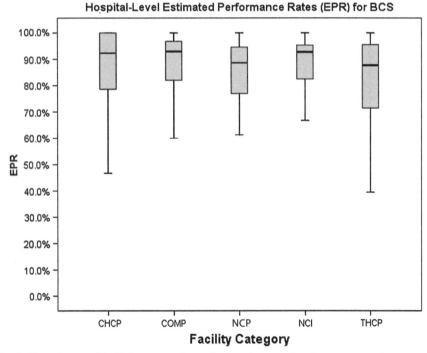

Fig. 6. Compliance with NQF measure for radiation therapy after breast-conserving surgery. BCS, breast-conserving surgery; CHCP, Community Hospital Cancer Program; COMP, Community Hospital Comprehensive Cancer Program; NCP, Network Cancer Program; THCP, Teaching Hospital Cancer Program.

Table 2
Facility category by surgery of the primary site, 2007 to 2008 (N = 294,452)

AJCC Stage		Surgery of the Primary Site	
		Breast-Conserving Surgery	**Mastectomy**
Stage 0	CHCP	77.6%	22.4%
	COMP	74.4%	25.6%
	THCP	74.1%	25.9%
	NCP	73.4%	26.6%
	NCI	69.1%	30.9%
Total		74.3%	25.7%
		46,400	16,021
Stage I	CHCP	75.0%	25.0%
	COMP	73.8%	26.2%
	THCP	73.6%	26.4%
	NCP	73.0%	27.0%
	NCI	70.3%	29.7%
Total		73.6%	26.4%
		87,454	31,303
Stage II (A,B)	CHCP	52.6%	47.4%
	COMP	51.1%	48.9%
	THCP	51.8%	48.2%
	NCP	51.6%	48.4%
	NCI	50.7%	49.3%
Total		51.5%	48.5%
		42,960	40,471
Stage III (A,B,C)	CHCP	23.8%	76.2%
	COMP	23.0%	77.0%
	THCP	24.2%	75.8%
	NCP	21.7%	78.3%
	NCI	27.1%	72.9%
Total		23.6%	76.4%
		7042	22,801

Abbreviations: CHCP, Community Hospital Cancer Program; COMP, Community Hospital Comprehensive Cancer Program; NCP, Network Cancer Program; THCP, Teaching Hospital Cancer Program.

at the time of diagnosis with breast cancer. Drs Nelson and Greene address breast conservation rates in the community setting in a separate article of this issue (**Fig. 7**).

Surgical treatment of the axilla was analyzed for stages I to III, stratified by nodal status (negative or positive) and category of the program. Patients treated with neoadjuvant therapy were excluded. The use of sentinel lymph node biopsy (SLN biopsy) and/or complete axillary lymph node dissection (ALND) was similar across all facility categories. Among node positive patients, complete axillary dissection was performed more frequently in mastectomy cases versus breast-conserving cases (18% vs 14%). This did not vary across program categories. In 7.5% of N0 patients, there was no axillary node sampling documented. Of this group, 55% were 70 years or older, a group for which axillary nodal staging might reasonably be omitted in many cases.[5,6] In addition, there was a higher percentage of patients with 1 or more comorbid condition (19%) in this group in comparison with the entire population (13%).

Among the node-negative patients, only 52% underwent SLN alone, ranging from 47% in community programs to 58% in NCI programs. Few N0 patients, perhaps 2%, might be predicted to have ALND because of the failure of SLN mapping, but

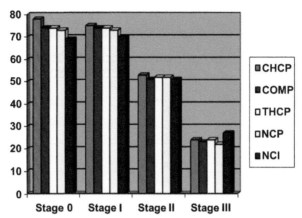

Fig. 7. Breast-conserving surgery rate by facility accreditation, 2007 to 2008 (N = 294,452). CHCP, Community Hospital Cancer Program; COMP, Community Hospital Comprehensive Cancer Program; NCP, Network Cancer Program; THCP, Teaching Hospital Cancer Program.

most patients with pathologic stage N0 would be expected to have SLN alone. This finding warrants further investigation, as does the surprisingly high incidence of ALND among node negative patients.

Among the node-positive patients, complete axillary dissection with or without sentinel node biopsy was done in about 88% of patients and only a sentinel node biopsy was performed in 10% of patients. Across all facility categories, SLN biopsy alone in node positive patients was twice as likely in breast conservation surgery than with mastectomy (14% vs 7%). It is likely that many of these cases involved patients with minimal disease identified in SLNs, not detected at the initial definitive surgical procedure. The percentage of node-positive patients who did not have ALND but did have axillary-specific radiation cannot be determined from the data examined. Patients with minimal disease seen in the SLNs may also have declined a return to the operating room. In addition, some recent reports support the use of sentinel node biopsy alone for patients with positive sentinel nodes.[6] The risk of axillary recurrence seems to be less.[7,8] It might be anticipated that in subsequent years, the percentage of patients with no axillary dissection for positive sentinel nodes will increase.

Five-Year Survival Data

Five-year all-cause mortality was analyzed for all patients with breast cancer diagnosed in 2003. Relative survival (adjusted to the general life expectancy of the US population by age, race, and gender) and multivariate analyses (adjusted for age, insurance type, race, income, tumor grade, comorbidity, and type of treatment) were reviewed. The survival rates were compared stage by stage among the program categories (**Figs. 8–11**).

For patients in stages I and III, the Community Hospital Cancer Programs had a statistically significantly lower likelihood of survival compared with NCI and academic programs. The interpretation of and conclusions drawn from these data should be made with caution because of the possible confounding factors. Community hospitals may be more likely to document mortality for their patients, who receive all their care locally, in typically smaller catchment areas and thus have a patient population that is comparatively more accessible for follow up. Nevertheless, some

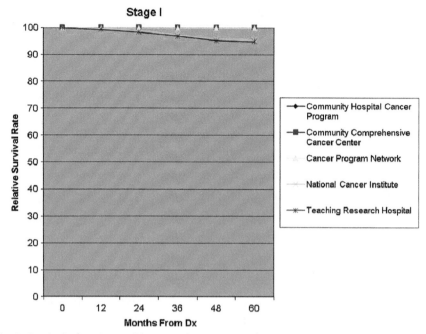

Fig. 8. Survival of patients with stage I breast cancer by CoC category. Dx, diagnosis.

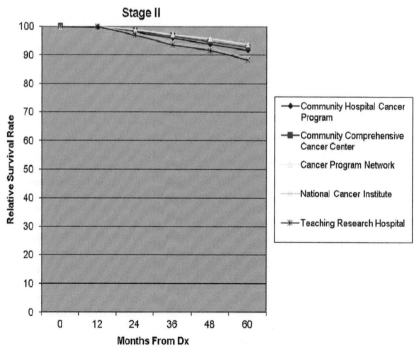

Fig. 9. Survival of patients with stage II breast cancer by CoC category. Dx, diagnosis.

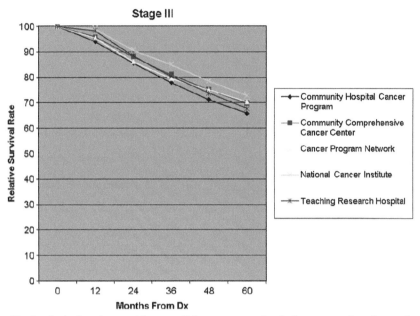

Fig. 10. Survival of patients with stage III breast cancer by CoC category. Dx, diagnosis.

variation in survival rate is not surprising, and the observed differences are not substantial. The larger facilities have higher volumes of patients with breast cancer, provide a wider and possibly more comprehensive range of services for patients, and are more likely to have high-volume, breast-focused surgeons or surgical

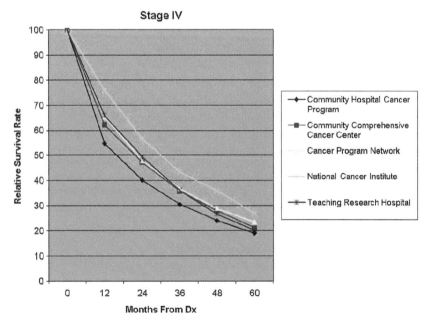

Fig. 11. Survival of patients with stage IV breast cancer by CoC category. Dx, diagnosis.

oncologists. The survival benefit, although not huge, could be related to the experience gained with higher volumes, use of more specialized services, and perhaps the implementation of more clinical trials. An article of this issue is devoted to a discussion of differences in outcome related to differences in hospital and physician volume.

Numerous previous reports have identified survival differences based on ethnicity, insurance type, and income level.[9–11] Results shown in this article seem to be consistent with these earlier reported findings. Even among patients in stage 0, there was a statistically significant lower likelihood of survival for Medicaid patients compared with those with private insurance or managed care. Across all other stages, survival was lower for Medicaid patients and Medicare patients, relative to private insurance or managed care. African Americans fared worse than white patients across all stages except stage 0. Such differences in survival rates imply possible disparities in treatment; however, no firm conclusions about treatment disparities are evident from these data.

In summary, our review of NCDB breast cancer treatment patterns and outcomes suggests that small incremental differences in breast-conserving surgery rates, extent of axillary surgery, and all-cause mortality for stages 0 and III breast cancer exist between the lower volume community cancer programs and the higher volume NCI and Teaching Hospital Cancer Programs. These differences could be explained by other confounding factors, but the impact of high-volume versus low-volume breast surgeons on some of these results cannot be excluded. In addition, the impact (if any) of CoC accreditation on minimizing or eradicating differences in care provided cannot be determined from these data.

The Community Breast Surgeon in 2010: What Is the Job Description?

The role of the breast surgeon has evolved over the last several decades. Previously, patients presented with palpable breast masses and were treated with mastectomy if the open biopsy and frozen-section analysis diagnosed breast cancer. There was no discussion of the possible options of therapy and no opportunity to educate women about their disease. Women were often in the hospital for a week after mastectomy, and support groups were conducted in the hospital during this recovery. Wanting more involvement in their own care, women demanded that there be some discussion of options and that consideration of breast-conserving surgery be part of that discussion. Screening mammograms began to be more common, and breast cancers were diagnosed at an earlier stage, thereby allowing more women to be able to save their breasts. Newer and more effective adjuvant treatment options also became available, and the survival rate of patients with breast cancer has improved annually since the early 1990s.

With these significant changes, the role of the breast surgeon has changed. The breast surgeon is most often the first physician to discuss with the patients the details of their diagnosis and the potential options of therapy available to them based on their individual situation. Breast cancer size, grade, axillary nodal status, hormone receptors, and her-2/neu expression are available and are part of the discussion. It is recommended that most breast cancers be diagnosed through a needle biopsy, so that those discussions can take place before any surgical procedure. Patients with larger tumors can be offered neoadjuvant chemotherapy or hormonal therapy. Surgeons must also be aware of and inform the patients about the available clinical trials.

The initial breast surgical consultation now involves review of the breast imaging, review of the pathology report, discussion of the options of therapy including systemic therapy and radiation therapy options, and recommendations for any neoadjuvant treatment. Referrals for fertility consultation and plastic surgery consultation are considered. Breast surgeons must be up-to-date on all aspects of breast cancer care, not just the surgical aspects. Written material provided from various sources may enhance but not replace a thorough discussion of the patient's case. Knowledge of national guidelines for treatment, such as National Comprehensive Cancer Network and American Society of Clinical Oncology guidelines, is important, as is knowledge of the latest research results that can guide the most effective therapy for that patient.

The surgeon works as a team with the radiologists and pathologists as well as the medical and radiation oncologists. Attention to details in the operating room such as orientation of all breast specimens, knowledge of sentinel node biopsies, use of ultrasound in the operating room to localize lesions and reduce the rate of positive margins, oncoplastic breast surgery techniques to improve cosmesis, referral to a genetic counselor, and involvement of plastic surgeons for contralateral procedures to provide breast symmetry are all important tools a breast surgeon uses. The breast surgeon's consultations with his or her patient can take several hours and occur for more than 1 day. Postoperatively, the breast surgeon must explain the pathology report fully and make appropriate referrals to medical and radiation oncologists. Multidisciplinary conferences are helpful to discuss imaging and histology among colleagues and to arrive at consensus regarding the appropriate next step for the patient.

Who Performs Breast Surgery in the United States?

Fifty percent of general surgeons perform a low volume of breast surgery (**Table 3**). In a study by Porter of 519 Canadian surgeons, 42% performed less than 2 breast cancer surgeries per month and 76% of surgeons surveyed took care of patients with breast cancer less than 25% of the time. Neuner,[12] in a study of 987 US surgeons, showed that about 50% of patients with breast cancer were cared for by doctors who performed 12 or fewer breast cancer surgeries over a 2-year period. Luther's[13] study found that 42% of surgeons performed less than 2 breast cancer surgeries per

Table 3 Breast cancer surgeon volume			
Author	Year	No. of Surgeons	Surgeon Volume
Porter[23]	2004	519	42% performed <2 breast cancer cases/month 76% of surgeons practice <25% breast surgery
Neuner[12]	2004	987	79% of physicians performed ≤12 operations/2 years, ~50% of patients with breast cancer
Waljee[19]	2007	318	34.5% of patients cared for by physicians <30% of practice is breast surgery 32.5% of patients cared for by physicians 30%–60% practice is breast surgery 33% patients cared for by physicians >60% practice is breast surgery
Luther[13]	2001	1320	42% of the physicians performed <2 breast cancer surgeries/year
Mikeljevic[14]	2003		Mean annual workload ≤29 new patients—27% of patients with breast cancer Mean annual workload 30–49 new patients—21% of patients with breast cancer Mean annual workload >50 new patients—52% of patients with breast cancer
McKee[18]	2002	125	50% of patients with breast cancer treated by low-volume surgeons

year. Mikeljevic,[14] at St James Hospital in Leeds, UK, has shown in a retrospective population-based study that patients with breast cancer treated by surgeons who treated less than 10 patients per annum had a statistically significant worse survival relative to patients treated by surgeons who treated more than 50 patients per annum (**Table 4**). The 5-year survival rate was 60% and 68%, respectively.[14] Sentinel node biopsy success rates have been associated with a higher volume of breast cancer cases.[15–17] Other studies have found no strong correlation between surgeon's volume of cases and patient outcomes.[18]

Several studies have indicated that patient satisfaction in the surgical decision-making process and in the surgeon-patient communication process was improved for patients cared for by breast-focused surgeons with higher volumes of cases.[19] Breast conservation rates may track with surgeon's volume of cases, 39% to 45% for low-volume surgeons versus 55% to 64% for higher volume surgeons.[13] Patients cared for by surgeons treating high volumes of patients with breast cancer are also more likely to be offered oncoplastic breast surgery techniques or breast symmetry operations,[20–22] breast reconstruction,[22–26] and clinical trial referral.[27]

High-volume surgeons may be more likely to adhere to national treatment guidelines and refer for multidisciplinary input.[12,14,28–34]

In addition to adhering to treatment guidelines, a breast surgeon must also be attuned to possible psychosocial challenges the patient may face. Patients may have language barriers, cultural barriers, or lack of insurance, which interfere with their ability to get a timely diagnosis and adequate care for their breast cancer diagnosis. Surgeons will require some support, particularly in the private practice environment, to better implement clinical trials. Any of these challenges adds to the complexity of the case management of the care of the patient with breast cancer. The surgeon becomes the primary caregiver during this time preoperatively and postoperatively, in addition to performing the surgical procedure.

Several countries have addressed the issues of oncology care, including breast cancer care, to better coordinate patient's care and provide a higher quality of care

Table 4
Breast surgeon volume and survival

Author	Year	Low-Volume Surgeons	Survival	High-Volume Surgeons
Mikeljevic[14]	2003	60%		68% 0.870
Golledge	2000	70%		75%
Chen[43]	2008	5-year survival 69.5% ≤44 cases/3 years	76.9% 45–200 cases/ 3 years	77.3% (>201 cases/3 years) 0.766
Allred	2006	92.1%	Survival differences decreased somewhat over time	95.9%
Gooiker	2010		Meta-analysis	0.80 HR
Bailie	2008			0.613 HR
Clayforth	2007			0.830 HR
Nattinger	2007			0.860 RR
Skinner	2003			0.84 RR

Abbreviations: HH, hazard ration; RR, relative risk.

with higher volume providers integrated in a system of care. In England, the Calman-Hine report, called "A Policy Framework for Commissioning Cancer Services," was published in April 1995 in response to varying treatments and outcomes for patients with cancer in the United Kingdom.[35] This report recommended significant reform of the United Kingdom's cancer services to improve outcomes and reduce inequities in the National Health Service cancer care. The primary recommendation was to concentrate the care of patients with cancer within site-specialized multidisciplinary teams. The reports showing the implementation of these recommendations are variable. However, where multidisciplinary teams had been established and specialist care for breast cancer had been implemented, there were quality improvements in areas such as adequate axillary node excision, recording of ER status, and use of hormonal therapy in ER-positive patients.[36–42]

Wales developed a breast-screening program called Breast Test Wales and has been analyzing the quality of care in their programs.[43]

In Germany, nationwide voluntary breast center certification and a collaborative network of breast centers have improved the indicators from report times between 2003 and 2007 as follows: preoperative diagnosis of breast cancer before diagnosis (58% in 2003 to 88% in 2007), appropriate endocrine therapy in hormone receptor–positive tumors (27% in 2003 to 93% in 2007), appropriate radiation therapy after breast-conserving surgery (20% in 2003 to 79% in 2007), and appropriate radiotherapy after mastectomy (8% in 2003 to 65% in 2007).[44,45]

In summary, the role of the modern breast surgeon has changed significantly from the former role with an operation and a little discussion. Today's breast surgeon must be knowledgeable about all the aspects of breast cancer and work together with a multidisciplinary team for the best outcomes for the patient. There is some evidence that both the surgical care and outcomes, use of appropriate referrals, multidisciplinary care, and perhaps even survival of patients with breast cancer are improved when patients are cared for by breast-focused surgeons who perform a high volume of breast surgeries.

Women with breast cancer should be offered the information and tools required to help them make informed choices about their care. Breast cancer surgeons are the first partner of the medical team whom patients encounter, and their information, recommendations, and surgical knowledge determine the course of treatment of their patients with breast cancer. This new role needs to be recognized, emphasized, and adequately compensated so that all women with breast cancer have the opportunity for the highest quality of care and potentially better outcomes and survival rates.

The American Society of Breast Surgeons and the Mastery of Breast Surgery Program

Numerous organizations have developed quality measures for breast cancer care, and although breast cancer care is multidisciplinary, many of the quality measures are the responsibility of the breast surgeon. However, there has not previously been a mechanism to collect current accurate performance data for breast surgery across the wide spectrum of practice environments.

The American Society of Breast Surgeons,[46] the primary leadership organization for general surgeons who treat patients with breast disease, is committed to continually improving the practice of breast surgery by serving as an advocate for surgeons who seek excellence in the care of patients with breast diseases. This mission is accomplished by providing a forum for the exchange of ideas and by promoting education, research, and the development of advanced surgical techniques. The society was formed in 1995 and currently has more than 2800 members. The demographics of the members reflect the diversity of breast care in the United States, with 54.4% private practice, solo or group; 5.3% academic; and 40.5% hospital based. The membership reflects a broad spectrum of breast care, with 31.5% of surgeons practicing exclusively breast surgery, 29% with more than 50% of their practice in breast surgery, and 21.4% with less than 50% of their practice in breast surgery.

The society recently developed the Mastery of Breast Surgery Program, a Continuing Quality Improvement Initiative. This program was developed in response to the urgent need for ongoing quality improvement in the practice of breast surgery. The goal of the program was to provide the surgeon with Web-based tools to document quality outcomes in patient care.

In December 2008, the society introduced the pilot phase of the program, which allowed individual surgeons to report and receive feedback on a limited number of quality measures for open surgical procedures for benign or malignant breast disease. The program was met with remarkable success, with more than 600 physicians registered to participate. In less than 2 years, more than 350 surgeons entered more than 60,000 cases by the time the Expanded Mastery Program was launched in June 2010.

The pilot program

The pilot phase of the mastery program was open to all surgeons who met the eligibility requirements, regardless of practice setting or volume of breast surgery. These requirements were based on recommendations of the Mastery of Breast Surgery Committee approved by the Board of Directors of the society, and represent minimum requirements for surgeons caring for patients with breast diseases. Board certification is required unless the surgeon has completed a breast surgery fellowship approved by American Society of Breast Disease, American Society of Breast Surgeons, Society of Surgical Oncology. Surgeons who were initially board certified but have not recertified because of a more focused practice were also eligible to apply.

Participation in the pilot program required a minimum of 8 hours of breast-specific American Medical Association Physician's Recognition Award category 1 continuing medical education (CME) credits within the previous year or 16 hours within 2 years before application. The CME credits can be obtained through a variety of courses, including education in breast surgical techniques, breast imaging, radiation physics, breast disease risk assessment, radiation or medical oncology, practice management for breast surgical practices, quality improvement, or public reporting of quality measures programs. Breast-specific CME can also be obtained through attendance at breast disease–specific meetings and other surgical meetings.

Participating surgeons were required to enter data for a minimum of 3 months on 3 specific quality measures on all open breast surgical procedures for both benign and malignant diseases. The simple, but critically important, surgeon-controlled quality measures are the following:

1. Was a needle biopsy performed to evaluate the breast lesion at some time before this procedure?[46–48]
2. Was the surgical specimen oriented?[46,47,49]
3. If a nonpalpable lesion was localized with image guidance, was there intraoperative confirmation of its removal?[47,50,51]

It was expected, and strongly encouraged, that the surgeon would continue to participate in the program by entering data on all of his or her open surgical breast cases. Ongoing participation maintains standing in the Mastery of Breast Surgery Program as it grows and develops new quality measures.

The Expanded Mastery Program

The Expanded Mastery Program, opened in June 2010, is intended to help surgeons document their clinical performance of breast procedures, both noninvasive and invasive, as well as their care of patients with breast cancer and those at risk for breast cancer. There is a risk assessment module, a percutaneous needle biopsy module, a breast cancer module, and a surgical module that has been qualified as a Physician Quality Reporting Initiative (PQRI) registry by the Centers for Medicare & Medicaid Services. There are 3 levels of participation in "Quality Measures," "Standard," and "PQRI," which define the required reporting fields in each module. The participant selects his or her level of participation and chooses which of the modules he or she wants to use depending on his or her desired reporting needs. The program is flexible and user friendly. The program has been designed to reflect the complexity of breast surgery, allowing for multiple patient encounters and data entry that may initially be incomplete. The program prompts the user regarding incomplete cases. Many participants delegate data entry to a member of their staff, particularly demographic and other data that will be familiar to office and clinical staff.

The user can change the levels of participation and the modules used at any time. The levels of participation are described below:

Risk assessment
- Standard level: Includes access to the Gail, Tamoxifen Benefit, Claus, and Myriad Mutation Prevalence Models.

Percutaneous procedures
- Standard level: Includes procedure, postprocedure, and follow-up information.
- Synoptic level: Includes all data fields in the standard level and adds the ability to create, save, and/or print a summary report.

Surgery
- Quality measures–only level: For participants who wish to track quality measures and not enter additional information.
- Standard level: Includes quality measures and adds data fields for the location of the procedure, indications, and pathologic condition. Formats data for downloading and submission to the American Board of Surgery (ABS) for Maintenance of Certification (MOC).
- PQRI level: Includes all data fields contained in the standard level plus required quality measures for data submission to PQRI.

Cancer
- Quality measures–only level: Includes quality measures with minimal clinical information.
- Standard level: Includes extensive cancer information with a staging module.
- Extended level: Includes components of the standard level plus quality measures–only level reporting.

Benefits of participation

It seems inevitable that surgeons will be required in the near future to document the quality of their work to obtain reimbursement. The ABS has recently recognized the Mastery of Breast Surgery Program as an acceptable quality initiative to meet the requirements of part 4 (Evaluation of Performance in Practice) for ABS MOC. The mastery program is a qualified 2010 PQRI registry for the Perioperative Measures Group. Eligible participants will receive incentive payments of 2% of the total estimate of allowed charges for covered professional services under Medicare part B in 2010 as long as the reporting requirements are met.

Participants in the mastery program will have access to their individual patient data through downloadable Excel spreadsheets. They will also be able to view their quality measures performance relative to other participants through reports that summarize quality measures for each module. The site is user friendly and encourages participants to provide feedback and suggestions.

All surgeons who successfully fulfill the requirements of continuous case reporting for a minimum of 3 months, complete the Mastery application, and have the appropriate level of CME credits will receive a printed certificate attesting to the participation in the Mastery of Breast Surgery Pilot Program. Now, the mastery program is free to members of the American Society of Breast Surgeons. Those surgeons interested in learning more about the mastery program can visit www.breastsurgeons.org and click on the Mastery of Breast Surgery icon. A username and password will be sent within 1 business day. Members' participation, comments, and feedback are vital to the program's success. Questions or comments should be directed to the Mastery of Breast Surgery Committee of the American Society of Breast Surgeons at masterybreastsurgery@breastsurgeons.org.

Measuring Outcomes in a Community Cancer Center Breast Program

The Helen F Graham Cancer Center experience

The Christiana Care Breast Center, part of the Helen F Graham Cancer Center in Newark, Delaware, was created in 2000 by a community hospital, in collaboration with a group of hospital-based radiologists, radiation oncologists, private practice surgeons, and medical oncologists (**Box 1**). The community had recognized a need to establish a centralized site for breast imaging and minimally invasive breast biopsies, for immediate surgical consultations for Breast Imaging Reporting and Data System (BIRADS) category 4 and 5 imaging findings, for a treatment planning tumor board, and for a multidisciplinary breast cancer clinic.

The first iteration of the Breast Center was an office shared by breast imaging and private practice breast surgeons. This space was soon outgrown, and the Breast Center moved to a new pavilion built to enlarge the Helen F Graham Cancer Center. The new Breast Center site included a dedicated breast-only MRI, breast ultrasound, female pelvic ultrasound, and separate offices for both private practice and hospital-employed breast surgeons. The cancer center in which the Breast Center is now housed includes hospital-employed genetic counselors, psychologists, rehabilitation medicine specialists, research nurses, nurse navigators, and hospital-based radiation oncologists. In the same pavilion are also offices of 2 large groups of private practice medical oncologists. Breast multidisciplinary clinics involving all these individuals and more are held weekly in the cancer center. The basic requirements for the "participating physicians" of Helen F Graham Cancer Center are summarized in **Box 1**.

Monitoring the quality of care

Goals on quality for the Breast Center are developed by a multidisciplinary team. One of the first goals was the development of a program for helping the patient with a "high-risk imaging result" navigate the path from mammogram through treatment. Nurses were hired by the Breast Center and trained in breast clinical examination and patient counseling. When a BIRADS category 4 or 5 mammogram or ultrasound is identified, the nurse and radiologist meet the patient in a private setting and explain the results to the patient. The patient is seen within 48 hours either by the surgeon of choice of the patient's primary care provider or by an "on-call" surgeon. The surgeons

---

Box 1
Multidisciplinary center participating physician's performance expectations for the Helen F Graham Cancer Center

Evidence as per the Cancer Research Department data source of placing a minimum of 4 patients on clinical trials each year.

Completion of the IRB mandatory ethics and HIPAA training courses.

Attends oncology seminars or conferences on a national, local/regional scale with CME documentation of 20 credits every 2 years in oncology-related topics.

Attends 66% of multidisciplinary conferences of the disease site on which the physician focuses.

Develops a publication record or record of presentations at national or regional oncology conferences.

Participates with case care managers (nurse navigators) with the multidisciplinary approach to cancer treatment and other supportive care services, such as psychology, genetic counseling, nutrition, and social services) as part of the multidisciplinary team.

Either has completed a fellowship in medical, surgical, or radiation oncology or is a general surgeon whose practice focuses on 1 or 2 surgical oncology disease sites.

Evidence of continuing commitment to oncology as demonstrated by activities such as oncologic teaching or research; involvement in activities of the CoC of the American College of Surgeons, American Society of Clinical Oncology, and/or NCI Cooperative Group Committees (ie, American College of Surgeons Oncology Group, Cancer and Leukemia Group B, Eastern Cooperative Oncology Group, Radiation Therapy Oncology Group, and National Surgical Breast and Bowel Project); a leadership role in hospital, state, or community cancer activities (such as Hospice, Wellness Group, Leukemia and Lymphoma Society, Delaware Breast Cancer Coalition, American Cancer Society, and Delaware Cancer Consortium), and membership in other oncologic societies.

"on call" for the Breast Center include breast surgeons employed by the cancer center and private practice "breast-focused" general surgeons who have satisfied the rigorous requirements for participation in the Helen F Graham Cancer Center. These requirements include attendance at tumor conference, accrual of patients into clinical trials, and evidence of scholarly activity (either published or through presentations).

The Breast Center tracks the timeline of care. Category 4 patients must have their definitive biopsy within 2 weeks, and category 5 patients must have theirs within 10 days. Performance on this indicator is presented to the multidisciplinary team (or breast Health Improvement Team). Work has begun to display a "dashboard" on the hospital Web site, displaying timelines from imaging to definitive biopsy or treatment for category 4 and 5 patients. Mammography (of which there are now more than 23,000 studies a year) is entirely digital. Results of biopsies for categories 4 and 5 are tracked for each mammographer. The category 4 or 5 positive predictive value (PPV) was 27% in 2008 and 22% in 2009 for 21,093 and 23,662 screening mammograms, respectively. The Breast Cancer Surveillance Consortium, an NCI partner, reported a PPV of 27.2% from 15,962 screening mammograms, with category 4 or 5 recommendations.[52] The percentages of screening studies placed in category 4 or 5 by each mammographer are also tracked and are also within the consortium guidelines.

The demographics of the screened population are monitored. When racial or other disparities are identified, the Breast Center works with the Helen F Graham cancer outreach staff to increase penetration into the underserved populations. The Breast Center works continually with the hospital's development office and with the Centers for Disease Control Screening for Life to obtain funds for care for indigent patients.

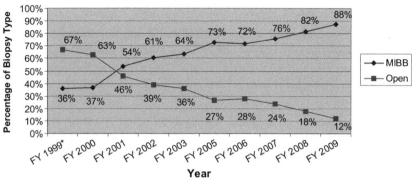

Fig. 12. Minimally invasive breast biopsy (MIBB) versus open breast biopsy.

The multidisciplinary team identified the need to reduce the number of open breast biopsies performed. An ongoing educational effort within the section of general surgery has resulted in a decrease in open breast biopsies from 67% of total to 12% of total over the past 10 years (**Fig. 12**). Another surgical quality indicator monitored is the percentage of patients with cancer requiring reexcision for close or involved margins. In an effort to reduce the number of reexcisions, the increased use of intraoperative ultrasound is encouraged, and a Faxitron (Lincolnshire, IL, USA) was purchased for the operating room for specimen radiography. The Faxitron image is viewed simultaneously, via the Picture Archiving and Communications System, by the operating surgeon and the mammographer. The surgeon and mammographer communicate while the patient is still on the table. The percentage of patients requiring a reexcision after segmental mastectomy was 33.9% in 2009, down from 49.3% in 2005 (**Fig. 13**).

The breast conservation versus mastectomy rate was also monitored for more than 20 general surgeons doing breast surgery at the Christiana Hospital. Six surgeons do 82% of the volume. In 2009, only 2 of these 6 surgeons would have fallen into the category of "high-volume" breast surgeons, using a cut-off of more than 106 cases a year to define that term. The most recent breast conservation rate is 66.7%. This rate has remained stable for almost a decade, even among the large group of surgeons who are less "breast focused." Arguably, the most important outcomes monitored by the Breast Center are in-breast-tumor-recurrence (IBTR) rate and regional and distant

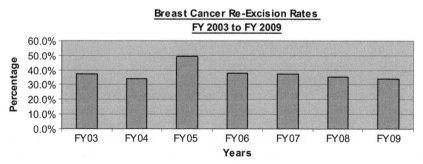

Fig. 13. Breast cancer reexcision rates, 2003 to 2009.

Table 5 Christiana care health system breast cancer recurrence rate (%) after breast conservation surgery						
	Recurrence Type					
Diagnosis Years	**None**	**In Breast**	**Regional**	**Distant**	**Never Disease Free**	**N**
1996–2000	86.8	3.5	1.1	5.0	3.7	1171
2001–2005	91.2	1.0	1.2	4.4	2.1	1606

recurrence rates, tracked by surgeon. The data are taken from the hospital tumor registry and are relayed back to the section of general surgery and the radiation oncology department. The overall IBTR rate at 5 years is 1% for patients who underwent breast conservation therapy (BCT) diagnosed from 2001 through 2005 (N = 1606). This rate is down from 3.5% for patients who underwent BCT diagnosed from 1996 to 2000 (N = 1606) (**Table 5**). According to Dr Solin,[53] national IBTR rates are approximately 5% at 10 years or 0.5% per year after treatment.

Dedicated breast tumor board

Two years ago, inspired by standards of the National Accreditation Program for Breast Centers, the authors initiated a breast-specific multidisciplinary tumor board for treatment planning. All cases are prospective. Case finding is done through the tumor registry. Most cases are presented by the surgeons.[54] In attendance and participating in discussion are medical oncologists, radiation oncologists, radiologists, pathologists, genetic counselors, research nurses, and nurse navigators. Referrals to genetic counseling have increased by 55% because of this conference, as has clinical trial accrual. Including all disease sites, the Helen F Graham Cancer Center has a 24% rate of NCI clinical trial accrual among analytical patients with cancer! The same phenomenon has been seen documented by others of significant numbers of cases where treatment plans are altered because of such a tumor board, including identification of additional sites of disease on review of images with radiology, and consideration of partial breast irradiation in patients appropriate for that modality according to American Society for Therapeutic Radiology and Oncology guidelines.[54,55]

In summary, the development of the Christiana Care Breast Center at the Helen F Graham Cancer Center is a testimony to the outcomes that can be accomplished at a community cancer center when there is real collaboration between a hospital and a multidisciplinary mix of employed and private practice providers. The overarching goals of this effort have been to improve the timeliness of care and the quality of the care, with the ultimate goal of improved outcomes for the patients. Areas of future concentration include collaborative work with the Cancer Center for improved survivorship support, increased clinical trial accrual, and increased use of the CoC's RQRS and similar tools for real-time tracking of actual progress through the steps of multidisciplinary breast cancer care.

SUMMARY

Evidence exists in the literature, summarized in this article, that high-volume breast surgeons have demonstrated better adherence to nationally recognized standards of surgical and multidisciplinary care; higher rates of use of breast-conserving surgery, sentinel node biopsy, and oncoplastic surgery; and in some cases better outcomes than have low-volume general surgeons. The complex and resource-intensive nature of a breast surgery practice has been illustrated.

However, a review of both outcomes and NQF breast cancer metrics as gleaned from the NCDB of the CoC reveals either no differences or small incremental differences between higher volume (NCI/academic/network) cancer programs and even the Community Hospital Cancer Programs, despite the fact that less than 50% of breast surgery in the community programs is done by high-volume breast surgeons. The absence of substantial differences in outcomes, despite significantly different volumes of patients with breast cancer seen annually at these programs and significant differences in individual breast surgeon volumes, suggests 1 of 2 conclusions. One is that surgeon volume is not a significant factor affecting treatment and outcome in breast cancer; however, it seems unlikely given the evidence in the literature alluded to previously. The second is that the standards of practice and cancer center infrastructure required for CoC accreditation, the multidisciplinary care requirements, the emphasis on national treatment guidelines, the continuous quality improvement process stipulated, and the metrics provided by the NCDB obviate the volume effects.

The impact of such continuous quality monitoring and improvement is demonstrated in the example of the breast cancer program at the Helen F Graham Cancer Center. Here, a mixture of faculty and private practice surgeons who have both high- and low-volume breast practices use these methods to optimize the care they provide and their patients' outcomes as measured by several quality indicators.

Continuous physician- and institution-specific performance evaluation is critical for identifying areas in which improvement is needed. The recent (September 7, 2010) release to the public of outcomes of coronary artery bypass graft procedures for 20% of US cardiac surgery programs should be a wake-up call for health care professionals.[56] We health care professionals are all officially on notice that the public will soon be demanding metrics for the comparison of both hospitals and physicians.

The CoC's CP3R and RQRS are an excellent beginning. More NQF measures need to be developed and added to the current CoC accountability and quality measures. More cancer programs need to participate in the accreditation programs of the CoC and the National Accreditation Program for Breast Centers so that they commit the required resources to the development and maintenance of appropriate infrastructure and quality measurement and improvement. In addition, more breast surgeons need to participate in programs such as the Mastery of Breast Surgery Program.

If the health care professionals do not participate fully in the creation, collection, and analysis of valid measures of the quality of care, then *invalid* metrics will be what the public and the third-party carriers see.

REFERENCES

1. Ferlay J, Shin HR, Bray F, et al. GLOBOCAN 2008, Cancer incidence and mortality worldwide: IARC CancerBase No. 10 [Internet]. Lyon (France): International Agency for Research on Cancer; 2010. Available at: http://globocan.iarc.fr. Accessed September 28, 2010.
2. Birkmeyer J. Measuring the quality of surgical care. J Am Coll Surg 2004;198:626–32.
3. Hillner BE. Hospital and physician volume or specialization and outcomes in cancer treatment: importance in quality of cancer care. J Clin Oncol 2000; 18(11):2327–40.
4. Schrag D. Influence of hospital procedure volume on outcomes following surgery for colon cancer. JAMA 2000;284(23):3028–35.
5. Martelli G, Miceli R, De Palo G, et al. Is axillary lymph node dissection necessary in elderly patients with breast carcinoma who have a clinically uninvolved axilla? Cancer 2003;97(5):1156–63.

6. Giuliano AE. Locoregional recurrences after sentinel lymph node dissection with or without axillary dissection in patients with sentinel lymph node metastases: the American College of Surgeons Oncology Group Z0011 randomized trial. Ann Surg 2010;252(3):432–3.

7. Hwang RF. Low locoregional failure rates in selected breast cancer patients with tumor-positive sentinel lymph nodes who do not undergo completion axillary dissection. Cancer 2007;110(4):723–30.

8. Jeruss JS. Axillary recurrence after sentinel node biopsy. Ann Surg Oncol 2005; 12(1):34–40.

9. DeSantis C. Disparities in breast cancer prognostic factors by race, insurance status, and education. Cancer Causes Control 2010;21(9):1445–50.

10. McKenzie F. Do lifestyle or social factors explain ethnic/racial inequalities in breast cancer survival? Epidemiol Rev 2009;31(1):52–66.

11. Gerend MA. Social determinants of Black-White disparities in breast cancer mortality: a review. Cancer Epidemiol Biomarkers Prev 2008;17(11):2913–23.

12. Neuner JM. Decentralization of breast cancer surgery in the United States. Cancer 2004;101:1323–9.

13. Luther SL. Physician practice volume and alternative surgical treatment for breast cancer in Florida. Health Serv Res 2001;36(6 Pt 2):166–79.

14. Mikeljevic SJ. Surgeon workload and survival from breast cancer. Br J Cancer 2003;89:487–91.

15. DuPont E. Learning curves and breast cancer lymphatic mapping: institutional volume index. J Surg Res 2001;97:92–6.

16. Johnson JM. Institutional learning curve for sentinel node biopsy at a community teaching hospital. Am Surg 2001;67:1030–3.

17. Cox CE. Learning curves for breast cancer sentinel lymph node mapping based on surgical volume analysis. J Am Coll Surg 2001;193:593–600.

18. McKee MD. Provider case volume and outcome in the evaluation and treatment of patients with mammogram-detected breast carcinoma. Cancer 2002;95(4):704–12.

19. Waljee JF. Patient satisfaction with treatment of breast cancer: does surgeon specialization matter? J Clin Oncol 2007;25:3694–8.

20. Hiotis K. Predictors of breast conservation therapy: size is not all that matters. Cancer 2005;103:892–9.

21. Nahabedian MY. Managing the opposite breast: contralateral symmetry procedures. Cancer J 2008;14:258–63.

22. Regano S. Oncoplastic techniques extend breast-conserving surgery to patients with neoadjuvant chemotherapy response unfit for conventional techniques. World J Surg 2009;33:2082–6.

23. Porter GA. Practice patterns in breast cancer surgery: Canadian perspective. World J Surg 2004;28:80–6.

24. Morrow M. Surgeon recommendations and receipt of mastectomy for treatment of breast cancer. JAMA 2009;302:1551–6.

25. Kollias J. Clinical impact of oncoplastic surgery in a specialist breast practice. ANZ J Surg 2008;78:225–6.

26. Zork NM. The effect of dedicated breast surgeons on the short-term outcomes in breast cancer. Ann Surg 2008;248:280–5.

27. Hofer TP. Does it matter where you go for breast cancer surgery? J Clin Oncol 2009;27(Suppl):15s [abstract 6504].

28. Sainsbury R. Does it matter where you live?: treatment variation for breast cancer in Yorkshire. The Yorkshire Breast Cancer Group. Br J Cancer 1995; 71:1275–8.

29. Rutgers EJ. Guidelines to assure quality in breast cancer surgery. Eur J Surg Oncol 2005;31:568–76.
30. Monaghan P. Breast cancer services—a population-based study of service reorganization. J Public Health (Oxf) 2005;27(2):171–5.
31. Katz SJ. Patterns and correlates of patient referral to surgeons for treatment of breast cancer. J Clin Oncol 2007;25:271–6.
32. Bouche G. Breast cancer surgery: do all patients want to go to high-volume hospitals? Surgery 2008;14:699–705.
33. Ma M. Breast cancer management: is volume related to quality? Clinical Advisory Panel. Br J Cancer 1997;75:1652–9.
34. Gilligan MA. Surgeon characteristics and variation in treatment for early-stage breast cancer. Arch Surg 2007;142:17–22.
35. Bickell NA. The quality of early-stage breast cancer care. Ann Surg 2000;232:220–4.
36. Richards MA. Variation in the management and survival of women under 50 years with breast cancer in the South East Thames region. Br J Cancer 1996;73:751–7.
37. McCarthy M. Is the performance of cancer services influenced more by hospital factors or by specialization? J Public Health (Oxf) 2008;30:69–74.
38. Allgood PC. Effects of specialization on treatment and outcomes in screen-detected breast cancers in Wales: cohort study. Br J Cancer 2006;94:36–42.
39. American Society of Breast Disease. Colloquium: ensuring optimal interdisciplinary breast care in the United States. American Society of Breast Disease [Online]. Available at: http://www.asbd.org. Accessed January 10, 2010.
40. The Expert Advisory Group on Cancer to the Chief Medical Officers of England and Wales. A policy framework for commissioning cancer services. Swyddfa Gymreig: Department of Health of Wales;1995.
41. Tataru D. Trends in the treatment of breast cancer on Southeast England following the introduction of national guidelines. J Public Health (Oxf) 2006;28:215–7.
42. Haward RA. The Calman-Hine report: a personal retrospective on the UK's first comprehensive policy on cancer services. Lancet Oncol 2006;794:336–46.
43. Chen CS. Does high surgeon and hospital surgical volume raise the five-year survival rate for breast cancer? a population-based study. Breast Cancer Res Treat 2008;110:340–56.
44. Rouse AM. Has Calman-Hine succeeded? Analysis of breast cancer procedure loads per consultant firm before and after the Calman-Hine report. Breast 2001;10:55–7.
45. Haward R. Breast cancer teams: the impact of constitution, new cancer workload, and methods of operations on their effectiveness. Br J Cancer 2003;89:15–22.
46. The American Society of Breast Surgeons. American Society of Breast Surgeons position statement: percutaneous needle biopsy for image detected breast abnormalities [online]. Available at: http://www.breastsurgeons.org/statements/mibb.php. Accessed June 12, 2006.
47. Silverstein MJ. Image-detected breast cancer: state of the art diagnosis and treatment. J Am Coll Surg 2005;201(4):586–97.
48. Brenner RJ. Stereotactic core-needle breast biopsy: a multi-institutional prospective trial. Radiology 2001;218(3):866–72.
49. Fleming FJ. Intraoperative margin assessment and re-excision rate in breast conserving surgery. Eur J Surg Oncol 2004;33(3):233–7.
50. Dixon JM. Specimen-orientated radiography helps define excision margins of malignant lesions detected by breast screening. Br J Surg 1993;80(8):1001–2.

51. Chagpar A. Intraoperative margin assessment reduces reexcision rates in patients with ductal carcinoma in situ treated with breast-conserving surgery. Am J Surg 2003;186(4):371–7.
52. Consortium, Breast Cancer Surveillance. Performance Benchmarks for Screening Mammography. Breast Cancer Surveillance Consortium [Online]. Available at: http://breastscreening.cancer.gov. Accessed September 21, 2010.
53. Solin LJ. Breast conservation treatment with radiation: an ongoing success story. J Clin Oncol 2010;28(5):709–11.
54. Newman EA. Changes in surgical management resulting from case review at a breast cancer multidisciplinary tumor board. Cancer 2006;107:2346–51.
55. Santoso JT. Tumor board in gynecologic oncology. Int J Gynecol Cancer 2004;14: 206–9.
56. Ferris TG, Torchiana DF. Public release of clinical outcomes data—online CABG report cards. N Engl J Med 2010;363:1593–5.

The National Accreditation Program for Breast Centers: Quality Improvement Through Standard Setting

David P. Winchester, MD[a,b,*]

KEYWORDS

• NAPBC • Breast centers • Accreditation • Standards

The breast center concept developed in response to a fragmented inefficient system to evaluate and manage patients with diseases of the breast. Historically, patients with breast complaints or abnormal results of imaging studies had to find their way through a complex environment, waiting for long periods to get appointments and receive reports. Silverstein,[1] some 4 decades ago, recognized these deficiencies and established the first free-standing breast center in the United States. This was to be the beginning of a major paradigm shift to address the needs of countless patients with benign and malignant diseases of the breast.

There is no reliable information about the number of breast centers, but one can estimate that the number is likely to be between 1300 and 1500. This estimate is based on the fact that the National Accreditation Program for Breast Centers (NAPBC) has received requests for information from more than 1400 parties. In addition, the Commission on Cancer (COC) of the American College of Surgeons (ACOS) currently accredits more than 1500 general cancer programs, and 98% of NAPBC-accredited breast centers and applicants are COC accredited.

Breast centers are not unique to the United States. For the past several years, European countries have developed multidisciplinary standards of care for patients

[a] University of Chicago Pritzker School of Medicine, Evanston Hospital, Walgreen Building, Suite 2507, 2650 Ridge Avenue, Evanston, IL 60201, USA
[b] American College of Surgeons, 633 North Saint Clair Street, Chicago IL 60611-3211, USA
* University of Chicago Pritzker School of Medicine, Evanston Hospital, Walgreen Building, Suite 2507, 2650 Ridge Avenue, Evanston, IL 60201.
E-mail address: dwinchester@facs.org

Surg Oncol Clin N Am 20 (2011) 581–586
doi:10.1016/j.soc.2011.01.011
1055-3207/11/$ – see front matter © 2011 Elsevier Inc. All rights reserved.

with diseases of the breast and a survey process to monitor compliance with the standards.[2] It is apparent that there is a growing global interest in organizing breast centers. The NAPBC has received inquiries from 20 countries around the world. The structure of a breast center would naturally depend on the resources, professional leadership, and government support in any particular country.

In the United States, the evaluation and management of patients with benign and malignant diseases of the breast are an enormous public health problem. It cannot be accommodated in a centralized, regional referral setting. Most care is delivered in a community setting. To assure the highest quality, there is a need for a multidisciplinary organized system with well-trained professionals. Fortunately, Disease of the breast disease is well taught in training programs, with many specialists possessing a major interest and experience in this field.

With this background, a need existed for assuring that these patients received well-organized competent care. The idea of an NAPBC to address this unmet need originated in the cancer programs at the ACOS. The Board of Regents of the college approved developmental funds in 2007. The college had experience and credibility in accrediting cancer, trauma, and bariatric centers; so it seemed natural to organize a breast center program. However, any new system proposal will, predictably, be met with some skepticism. The NAPBC strongly believed that this was the right thing to do and has prevailed.

A multidisciplinary Board of Directors, consisting of 32 members from 16 national organizations/societies, was organized and has continued to shape the NAPBC (**Box 1**). The NAPBC Mission Statement states that "The NAPBC is a consortium of national, professional organizations dedicated to the improvement of the quality of care and monitoring of outcomes of patients with diseases of the breast. This mission

---

Box 1
NAPBC member organizations

American Board of Surgery

American Cancer Society

American College of Surgeons

American Society of Breast Disease

American Society of Breast Surgeons

American Society of Clinical Oncology

American Society of Plastic Surgeons

American Society for Radiation Oncology

Association of Cancer Executives

Association of Oncology Social Work

College of American Pathologists

National Cancer Registrars Association

National Consortium of Breast Centers

National Society of Genetic Counselors

Oncology Nursing Society

Society of Surgical Oncology

Members-at-Large

is pursued through standard-setting, scientific validation and patient and professional education."

The NAPBC Board of Directors defined 17 essential components of evaluation and management every patient with disease of the breast should receive (**Box 2**). To broaden the accessibility of patients to centers without compromising any step in the continuum, accredited centers may provide services on-site or refer to nearby locales for services they may not have, such as genetic counseling.

Likewise, the board defined 27 evidence- and consensus-based standards that accredited centers had to meet (**Box 3**). There are 3 mandatory standards in the pre-application that validate a center's eligibility for survey: (1) the organizational structure of the breast center gives the breast program leadership (BPL) responsibility and accountability for provided breast center services; (2) the BPL establishes, monitors, and evaluates the interdisciplinary breast cancer conference frequency, attendance, prospective case presentations, including the American Joint Committee on Cancer (AJCC) staging, and discussion of nationally accepted guidelines; and (3) after a diagnosis of breast cancer, the patient management is conducted by an interdisciplinary team. The team members are either board certified or in the process of board certification.

NAPBC accreditation is granted only to those centers that have voluntarily committed to provide the best in the diagnosis and treatment of breast cancer and are able to comply with the established NAPBC standards. Each center must undergo a rigorous evaluation and review of its performance and compliance with the NAPBC standards. To maintain accreditation, centers must undergo an on-site review every 3 years. To be scheduled for survey, each center must complete an electronic survey application record.

Box 2
NAPBC components

1. Imaging
2. Needle biopsy
3. Pathology
4. Interdisciplinary conference
5. Patient navigation
6. Genetic evaluation and management
7. Surgical care
8. Plastic surgery consultation/treatment
9. Nursing
10. Medical oncology consultation/treatment
11. Radiation oncology consultation/treatment
12. Data management
13. Research
14. Education, support, and rehabilitation
15. Outreach and education
16. Quality improvement
17. Survivorship program

Box 3
NAPBC standards

Center leadership

Standard 1.1. Level of responsibility and accountability[a]

Standard 1.2. Interdisciplinary breast cancer conference[a]

Standard 1.3. Evaluation and management guidelines

Clinical management

Standard 2.1. Interdisciplinary patient management[a]

Standard 2.2. Patient navigation

Standard 2.3. Breast conservation

Standard 2.4. Sentinel node biopsy

Standard 2.5. Breast cancer surveillance

Standard 2.6. Breast cancer staging

Standard 2.7. Pathology reports

Standard 2.8. Diagnostic imaging

Standard 2.9. Needle biopsy

Standard 2.10. Ultrasonography

Standard 2.11. Stereotactic core needle biopsy

Standard 2.12. Radiation oncology

Standard 2.13. Medical oncology

Standard 2.14. Nursing

Standard 2.15. Support and rehabilitation

Standard 2.16. Genetic evaluation and management

Standard 2.17. Education resources

Standard 2.18. Reconstructive surgery

Standard 2.19. Evaluation and management of benign breast disease

Research

Standard 3.1. Clinical trial information

Standard 3.2. Clinical trial accrual

Community outreach

Standard 4.1. Education, prevention, and early detection programs

Professional education

Standard 5.1. Breast center staff education

Quality improvement

Standard 6.1. Quality and outcomes

[a] NAPBC Critical Standards.

Table 1
NAPBC site visit agenda

Agenda Item	Time Required
Time for the surveyor to speak/meet with the breast center leadership and key staff responsible for various aspects of the program and to assess the center's compliance with each standard through review of the survey application	1–2 h
Time for chart review	2 h
Tour of center	30 min
To attend a breast conference (survey should be held on a day when a conference is scheduled)	1 h
Surveyor private time to compile recommendations	30 min
Summation meeting with the breast center team	30 min

The site visit agenda is summarized in **Table 1**. The NAPBC has 50 physician surveyors trained annually. The survey is conducted by 1 surveyor. Twenty breast cancer charts, stage I, II, or III, are selected by the surveyor to validate compliance. The center provides an additional 10 benign cases, including atypical ductal or lobular hyperplasia, for review. The accreditation award is based on the matrix described in **Table 2**.

The NAPBC has accredited several different breast center models. A community-based group of private practice specialists, in a center with or without walls, have organized themselves and met the standards. The most common accredited breast center models are found in nonteaching hospitals or academic/teaching hospitals.

NAPBC-accredited centers experience several benefits: (1) a model for organizing and managing a breast center to ensure multidisciplinary, integrated, and comprehensive breast care services; (2) internal and external assessments of breast center performance based on recognized standards; (3) recognition as having met performance measures for high-quality breast care established by national breast care organizations; (4) national recognition and public promotion; (5) participation in a national breast cancer database to report patterns of care and effect quality improvement; and (6) access to breast center comparison benchmark reports containing national aggregate data and individual center data to assess patterns of care and outcomes relative to national norms.

Table 2
Accreditation award matrix based on compliance with 27 standards

3-y/Full Accreditation	3-y Contingency Accreditation	Accreditation Deferred
90% or more (24 or more) of the eligible standards are met. Full accreditation awarded with recommendation for improvement in any deficient standards within a 12-mo period.	Less than 90% and greater than 75% (between 20 and 24) of the eligible standards are met. Full accreditation withheld until correction of deficient standards is documented within a 12-mo period.	Less than 75% (less than 20) of the eligible standards are met. Full accreditation deferred until correction of deficient standards and resurvey in 12 mo.

The NAPBC has experienced significant success. The first center was surveyed in late December 2008. As of February 2011, the NAPBC has accredited 270 centers in 41 states, with another 115 scheduled for survey. The NAPBC recently conducted a survey of 160 accredited centers. More than 80% reported that preparation for their site visit resulted in enhanced organization and coordination of their center; 80% reported using their tumor registry to complete the application for survey; 75% to 80% required 3 to 9 months for survey readiness; and 70% implemented program component changes in their centers.

Regarding the performance of accredited centers, standard 2.3 states that a proportion of at least 50% of all patients diagnosed with early-stage breast cancer (stage 0, I, or II) are offered and/or treated with breast-conserving surgery, and compliance is evaluated annually by the breast program leadership. Of these patients, 65% have undergone breast-conserving surgery and 35% mastectomy.

The ultimate value of the NAPBC must be based on data-driven improvement in compliance with quality measures.

Accredited programs have been held accountable for the 3 National Quality Forum accountability measures as summarized in the Breast Center Standards Manual of the NAPBC[3]: (1) radiation therapy is administered within 1 year (365 days) of diagnosis for women younger than 70 years receiving breast-conserving surgery for breast cancer; (2) combination chemotherapy is considered or administered within 4 months (120 days) of diagnosis for women younger than 70 years with AJCC T1c, stage II or III hormone receptor–negative breast cancer; and (3) tamoxifen or third-generation aromatase inhibitor is considered or administered within 1 year (365 days) of diagnosis for women with AJCC T1c, stage II or III hormone receptor–positive breast cancer.

Measures to be implemented in 2011 include the following: (1) the percentage of patients presenting with AJCC stage 0, I, II, or III disease who undergo surgical excision/resection of a primary breast tumor having a needle biopsy to establish the diagnosis of cancer preceding surgical excision/resection and (2) radiation therapy is considered or administered within 1 year (365 days) of diagnosis for women with AJCC stage III breast cancer undergoing mastectomy with 4 or more positive regional lymph nodes. The NAPBC is in the process of defining the most efficient methods of data collection for both NAPBC-accredited programs associated with the COC and independent practices.

REFERENCES

1. Silverstein MJ. The Van Nuys Breast Center. The first free-standing multidisciplinary breast center. Surg Oncol Clin N Am 2003;9:159–76.
2. Blamey RW, Cataliotti L. EUSOMA accreditation of breast units. Eur J Cancer 2006; 42:1331–7.
3. NAPBC. Breast center standards manual. Chicago (IL): American College of Surgeons; 2008.

Improving Uniformity of Care for Colorectal Cancers Through National Quality Forum Quality Indicators at a Commission on Cancer–accredited Community Based Teaching Hospital

Dean P. Pappas, MD[a,b], Jules E. Garbus, MD[a,b],
Martin Feuerman, MS[c], William P. Reed, MD[a,b],*

KEYWORDS

- Colon cancer • Rectal cancer • Preoperative radiation • Nodes

Winthrop-University Hospital is a 591 bed community based teaching hospital affiliated with the State University of New York at Stony Brook (SUNY-SB). The hospital provides clinical clerkships and fourth year electives for students from SUNY-SB and will soon become a clinical campus of the medical school with full responsibility for the final 2 years of education for a cohort of these students. The hospital offers independent residencies in internal medicine, obstetrics-gynecology, pathology, pediatrics, and radiology, and has integrated residencies with SUNY-SB in general surgery and orthopedics. Fellowships are available in many medical and pediatric subspecialties, as well as in colorectal surgery and vascular surgery.

Most faculty members, particularly in surgery, are community physicians. In General Surgery, there are 40 practicing surgeons, of whom 9 are full time. Eight of the general

The authors have nothing to disclose.

[a] State University of New York at Stony Brook, NY 11794-8191, USA

[b] Department of Surgery, Winthrop-University Hospital, 259 First Street, Mineola, NY 11501, USA

[c] Health Outcomes Research-Biostatistics, Winthrop-University Hospital, 259 First Street, Mineola, NY 11501, USA

* Corresponding author. Department of Surgery, Winthrop-University Hospital, 259 First Street, Mineola, NY 11501.

E-mail address: wreed@winthrop.org

Surg Oncol Clin N Am 20 (2011) 587–596
doi:10.1016/j.soc.2011.01.013
1055-3207/11/$ – see front matter © 2011 Published by Elsevier Inc.

surgonc.theclinics.com

surgeons have also been fellowship trained in colorectal surgery and all of these are community surgeons. Most of the colorectal surgeons work for 1 of 2 groups, but there are solo practitioners as well, which leads to a diversity of practice settings and styles for those surgeons engaged in the resection of colorectal cancers.

Winthrop has had a cancer program accredited by the Commission on Cancer (COC) since 1966. The COC began to provide information to its accredited programs in 2005 on the degree to which these programs were adhering to standards of care associated with best outcomes. Initially this program, called the Cancer Program Practice Profiles Reports (CP3R), focused on the use of adjuvant chemotherapy after resection of node positive (stage III) colon cancer. Data from the National Cancer Data Base (NCDB) on the use of chemotherapy after resection of node positive colon cancer was reported back to each accredited center with a ranking of its performance as concordant if the center was in the top 25% of centers in the use of chemotherapy, or nonconcordant if it was in the bottom 75%. If they were nonconcordant, centers were provided with registry accession numbers for the patients who did not receive the recommended therapy to enable them to review and update their records. Winthrop's data, at the time of initial reporting, was concordant for this measure, (**Tables 1** and **2**) so there was little incentive to change treatment patterns.

Beginning in 2008, the COC expanded its CP3R measures to 6, 4 of which were endorsed by the National Quality Forum (NQF). The new measures focused on 3 parameters in the treatment of breast cancer and 3 parameters in the treatment of colorectal cancer. For colorectal cancer, the measures continued the assessment of chemotherapy use for stage III colon cancers and added an assessment of the number of lymph nodes removed during resection of colon cancers and the use of radiation in the treatment of rectal cancer. These added measures provided an opportunity to study the quality of care provided by surgeons caring for colorectal cancer at our institution and form the basis for this report.

MATERIALS AND METHODS

Data on the use of radiation for rectal cancer and the numbers of lymph nodes removed during colon resection for treatment of colon cancer for the years 2004 to 2007 were obtained from the CP3R information provided online to Winthrop by the NCDB (**Fig. 1**). Review of the NCDB CP3R data on the use of radiation for patients less than 80 years of age with T4N0M0 or stage III rectal cancer showed that all 12

Table 1
Winthrop-University Hospital cancer program practice profile reports (CP3R) for rectum cancers diagnosed 2004 to 2007

	Performance Rates and Reported Cases				
	2004	2005	2006	2007	All
Radiation therapy is considered or administered within 6 mo (180 d) of diagnosis for patients <80 y with clinical or pathologic AJCC T4N0M0 or stage III receiving surgical resection for rectal cancer:					
Estimated performance rates (%)	100	100	100	100	100
Performance rate (numerator/ denominator)	4/4	1/1	4/4	3/3	12/12
Total number of rectum cancer cases reported to NCDB	25	27	31	19	102

Abbreviation: AJCC, American Joint Commission for Cancer.

Table 2
CP3R for colon cancers diagnosed 2004 to 2007

	Performance Rates and Reported Cases				
	2004	2005	2006	2007	All
At least 12 regional lymph nodes are removed and pathologically examined for resected colon cancer:					
Estimated performance rates (%)	73.3	88.9	73.9	85.4	79.9
Performance rate (numerator/ denominator)	44/60	40/45	34/46	41/48	159/199
Total number of colon cancer cases reported to NCDB	142	112	104	124	482

eligible patients at Winthrop for the years 2004 to 2007 were treated with radiation within the 180 days of diagnosis considered appropriate. However, only 12 of 102 patients with rectal cancer during these 4 years fitted the eligibility criteria for radiation treatment. Treating physicians considered that greater numbers of patients who had rectal cancers were receiving radiation and that further scrutiny of the registry data was in order.

Review of the NCDB CP3R data on the numbers of nodes harvested during resection of colon cancer for the years 2004 to 2007 showed, on average for the 4 years, that 79.9% of patients had at least 12 nodes removed. The year-to-year average varied from 73.3% for 2004 to 88.9% for 2005. Although these percentages seemed good, our surgeons did not think that they were as high as they would like them to be. Furthermore, the effect on patient care was uncertain, because the NCDB numbers did not indicate the frequency of nodal involvement for those patients having fewer than 12 nodes removed. If all these patients had negative nodes and did not receive chemotherapy for this reason, the potential effect on outcome would be greater than if the reverse were true.

To better assess the implications of the CP3R data provided by the NCDB, registry abstracts and charts were reviewed for rectal and colon cancer cases for the years 2004 to 2007. Additional colon cases for the years 2008 and 2009 were examined for more current information on the harvest of nodes during colon resection.

RECTAL CANCER ALGORITHM-PART I

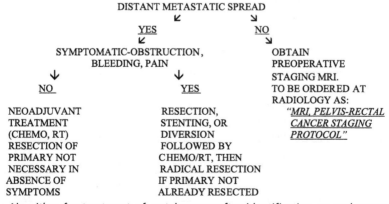

Fig. 1. Algorithm for treatment of rectal cancer after identification on endoscopy, diagnostic confirmation by biopsy, and computed tomography evaluation for metastatic spread.

To evaluate whether deficiencies in nodal harvest were related to the use of laparo-scopic colon resection, we performed a retrospective chart review of all colon resec-tions, both laparoscopic and open, performed for cancer for the years 2008 and 2009. Parameters analyzed included specimen length, mesenteric length and height (**Table 3**), and the number of harvested lymph nodes (**Table 4**). The rank-sum test was used to compare groups, because the data were skewed. The Fisher exact test was used to find differences in rates between the groups having 12 or more nodes examined (**Table 5**).

RESULTS
Rectal Cancer

Review of the cases of rectal cancer at Winthrop for the years 2004 to 2007 showed that all patients who met the criteria established by the NCDB for adjuvant radiation within 6 months of diagnosis did receive this treatment in a timely manner (see **Tables 1** and **2**). In addition, there were 17 patients who received radiation as adjuvant treatment to resection who fell outside the eligibility criteria of the NCDB, either because they were older than 80 years or had tumors that were earlier than stage III or T4. Two of the 17 patients treated with adjuvant radiation were older than 80 years. Most additional cases did not meet the criteria because the tumors were less advanced than T4 or stage III, or could not be staged after preoperative radiation.

Radiation was given preoperatively to 21 of the 29 patients in this series, including most of those (13/17) who failed to meet the criteria for radiation treatment by NCDB (**Table 6**). A possible explanation for these cases not meeting the NCDB criteria for radiation is that they were downstaged by the treatment and that their postirradiation stage no longer qualified them for this treatment. Although such downstaging could be considered a desirable effect that requires no remedial action, 2 patients were radi-ated after surgery for lesions that staged them pathologically as stage 0 or 1. Radiation in such circumstances would likely represent overtreatment and needs to be exam-ined in greater detail.

Colon Cancer

Review of the cases of colon cancer resected at Winthrop for the years 2004 to 2007 showed that 79.9% of specimens on average contained 12 or more nodes. Operative notes and pathology reports for 2007, the last year of NCDB reporting, were obtained for those cases in which fewer than 12 nodes were obtained to see whether any

Table 3 Colon cancer resections 2008 to 2009: mean gross specimen dimensions				
	Laparoscopic Right Colectomy (n = 43)	Open Right Colectomy (n = 59)	Laparoscopic Left Colectomy (n = 26)	Open Left Colectomy (n = 68)
	Mean	Mean	Mean	Mean
Total length (cm)	27.4	35.5	22.5	23.5
Ileal length (cm)	6.46	8.54	NA	NA
Colon length (cm)	21.2	27.3	NA	NA
Mesenteric length (cm)	21.8	26.9	22.3	22.4
Mesenteric width (cm)	5.88	7.15	6.1	6.6

Table 4									
Colon cancer resections 2008 to 2009: nodal harvest									
	Lap Surgery			Open Surgery			Both Methods		
Side	N	Mean	SD	N	Mean	SD	N	Mean	SD
Right	43	20.5[a]	8.9	59	20.6[a]	9.2	102	20.6[a]	9.0
Left	26	13.8	8.3	68	17.0	7.9	94	16.1	8.1
Both Sides	69	18.0	9.2	127	18.7	8.7	196	18.4	8.8

Abbreviations: Lap, laparoscopic; SD, standard deviation.
[a] Right side average total nodes significantly higher than left ($P<.05$).
All other differences are not significant statistically.

patterns in the deficient cases could be identified and to determine whether the failure to identify sufficient numbers of nodes would be likely to affect outcome. In addition, colon specimens with fewer than 12 lymph nodes from 2008 and 2009 were reviewed.

There were a total of 26 cases for the years 2007, 2008, and 2009 out of 150 eligible resections (17%) in which fewer than 12 nodes were obtained. On review of the pathology reports, 2 cases had at least 12 nodes removed. Of the remaining 24 cases, 8 (one-third) had positive nodes. Because chemotherapy would have been recommended for these patients as a matter of course, the therapeutic effect of having removed insufficient numbers of nodes is likely to have been negligible. Sixteen patients with fewer than 12 nodes removed were node negative. In these cases, the nodes removed ranged from 2 to 11. Although the effect on outcome of removing only 10 or 11 nodes (7/16 cases) may be small, there is reason to be concerned that those patients having fewer than 10 nodes removed (9/16 cases) may have been node positive. Of the 16 patients who were N0 and had fewer than 12 nodes removed, 9 (56%) had their resections performed laparoscopically. The number of nodes removed laparoscopically ranged from 2 to 11 (mean 6.8). In contrast, open colectomy provided 4 to 11 nodes (mean 8.6).

A more detailed analysis of open versus laparoscopic colon resection based on the review of pathology reports on all cases from 2008 and 2009 is shown in **Tables 1** and **2**. There were 102 right hemicolectomies in this time period, of which 43 were performed laparoscopically and 59 open. There were 94 left hemicolectomies, of which 26 were performed laparoscopically and 68 open. For the right-sided resections, node harvest was similar for the 2 groups (20.5 nodes per case for laparoscopic cases vs 20.6 for open, $P = .94$), although the laparoscopic resections produced shorter specimens (21.2 cm laparoscopic vs 27.3 cm open) and smaller mesenteric volumes

Table 5						
Colon cancer resections 2008 to 2009: total nodes. Percentage of cases with 12 or more nodes						
	Lap Surgery		Open Surgery		Both Methods	
Side	N	PCT (%)	N	PCT (%)	N	PCT (%)
Right	43	90.7[a]	59	86.4	102	88.2[a]
Left	26	69.2	68	76.5	94	74.5
Both Sides	69	82.6	127	81.1	196	81.6

Abbreviation: PCT, percent.
[a] Right side percentage significantly higher than left ($P<.05$).
All other differences are not significant statistically.

			RT/No Resection	RT +		Met NCDB	Met NCDB
Year	Total Cases	Total RT	(Stage 4 or Age)	Resection	Preop RT	Criteria	+ Preop RT
2004	23	13	3	10	7	4	2
2005	29	9	3	6	4	1	1
2006	29	11	4	7	4	4	2
2007	25	9	3	6	6	3	3
Totals	106	42	13	29	21	12	8

Table 6
Winthrop-University Hospital rectal cancers 2004 to 2007

Abbreviations: Preop, preoperative; RT, radiation therapy.

(length times width: 128.18 cm^3 laparoscopic vs 192.33 cm^3 open). For the left-sided colon resections, the number of harvested nodes was lower for the laparoscopic group (laparoscopic 13.8 cm^3 vs open 17 cm^3, P = .12), although the specimen sizes were not different for the 2 groups. The difference in nodal harvest suggested that the laparoscopic approach was less effective in retrieving nodes for left-sided lesions, but the difference was not statistically significant. There was a significant difference in the number of nodes retrieved, in favor of right-sided procedures ($P<.05$), no matter which surgical approach was used. This finding was confirmed by the comparison of the percentage of cases having 12 or more nodes removed among the different groups (see **Table 5**). Again, there was no significant difference between the surgical approach used (90.7% vs 86.4%, laparoscopic vs open approach for right colon procedures, P = .55, and 69.2% vs 76.5%, laparoscopic vs open approach for left colon procedures, P = .60) in the percentages of cases with 12 or more nodes removed, but a significantly better retrieval (88.2% vs 74.5%, $P<.05$) for right-sided procedures was obtained.

PROPOSED CORRECTIVE ACTIONS
Rectal Cancer

Most of the patients who did not meet the NCDB criteria for adjuvant treatment with radiation for rectal cancer, failed because of having a lower stage on the postradiation resected specimen (I or IIA) than that required to justify this treatment (IIB, IIC, or III). Because National Cancer Center Network (NCCN) guidelines for preoperative chemoradiation are less restrictive than those of the NCDB, recommending such treatment of patients with stage IIA disease (T3N0) as well as for those with T4 lesions and stage III disease,[1] the use of preoperative radiation may have been appropriate for some of these earlier-stage patients on this basis alone.[1] For other patients, it is likely that they would have met the treatment parameters had they been adequately staged before treatment was undertaken. A better system of establishing and documenting pretreatment staging was needed.

With this in mind, the Colorectal Disease Site Group of the Cancer Committee has developed a Rectal Cancer Staging Protocol to enhance the pretreatment staging of rectal cancer at Winthrop. The protocol consists of using magnetic resonance imaging (MRI) of the pelvis for both localization and staging. Once a lesion is identified on endoscopy, the diagnosis of adenocarcinoma is confirmed on biopsy, and the absence of distant disease is confirmed on computed tomography scan (see **Fig. 1**), an MRI, with focused pelvic views and enhancement, is performed for the purpose of confirming location and documenting stage (**Fig. 2**). Tumors above the

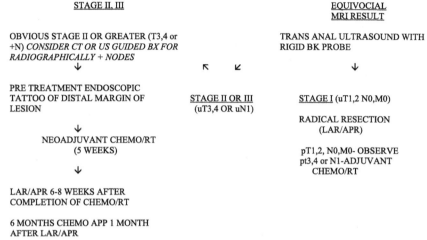

RECTAL CANCER ALGORITHM-PART II

OBTAIN PREOPERATIVE STAGING MRI. TO BE ORDERED AT WUH RADIOLOGY AS
"MRI, PELVIS-RECTAL CANCER STAGING PROTOCOL"

STAGE II, III   EQUIVOCIAL
                                                 MRI RESULT

OBVIOUS STAGE II OR GREATER (T3,4 or   TRANS ANAL ULTRASOUND WITH
+N) *CONSIDER CT OR US GUIDED BX FOR*   RIGID BK PROBE
RADIOGRAPHICALLY + NODES
          ↓   ↖   ↙   ↓

PRE TREATMENT ENDOSCOPIC
TATTOO OF DISTAL MARGIN OF   STAGE II OR III   STAGE I (uT1,2 N0,M0)
LESION   (uT3,4 OR uN1)

                                                    RADICAL RESECTION
          ↓   (LAR/APR)
NEOADJUVANT CHEMO/RT
     (5 WEEKS)   pT1,2, N0,M0- OBSERVE
                                                    pt3,4 or N1-ADJUVANT
          ↓   CHEMO/RT

LAR/APR 6-8 WEEKS AFTER
COMPLETION OF CHEMO/RT

6 MONTHS CHEMO APP 1 MONTH
AFTER LAR/APR

Fig. 2. Steps in the treatment of stage I to III rectal cancer.

sacral promontory are to be classified as colonic and not considered for preoperative chemoradiation. Tumors below the promontory, within the confines of the pelvis, are to be classified as rectal and considered for preoperative treatment as appropriate for their stage. Stage is to be determined on MRI, if possible. If the T or N stage is not clear by MRI, patients are referred for transanal ultrasound. Those patients with T1N0M0 or T2N0M0 tumors by ultrasound undergo resection. More deeply invasive tumors and those with lymph node involvement undergo preoperative treatment with chemoradiation after the distal margin of the lesion is tattooed to assure that it can be identified at the time of later resection. Records are monitored to assure compliance with the protocol and confirm whether lower-stage lesions treated with radiation are a result of the treatment or caused by protocol violations. In all cases, the pretreatment stage is recorded and reported to the registry to be tracked as the clinical or working stage.

We created this algorithm to ensure that the treating physicians at Winthrop adhere to the NCCN guidelines as closely as possible. Recent data have shown that MRI may be superior to transanal ultrasound (TAUS) for the pretreatment staging of rectal cancer.[2–7] Moreover, Winthrop has state-of-the-art MRI as well as a dedicated staff that works closely with the Colorectal Disease Site Group. The MRI is located on site, whereas the TAUS system is off site, in a private practice office. As a consequence, MRI is more readily available. It is also less dependent on the user. The rectal MRI protocol requires the attending radiologist to be present during the study, to review the images in real time, and to administer rectal contrast if needed. An intra-anal coil is not used. If the study is inconclusive, TAUS can then be performed by the colorectal surgeon trained in this area. Currently, this individual has more than a decade of rectal ultrasound experience.

Colon Cancer

The identification of fewer than 12 lymph nodes in 24 colon cancer cases in the years 2004 to 2007 is in 2 categories. One-third of the patients (8) had from 1 to 11 tumor-containing lymph nodes in from 6 to 11 nodes harvested. Because these patients would have had chemotherapy recommended because of their node positivity, the main effect of their having too few nodes removed is on the accuracy of reported pathologic tumor-node-metastasis staging rather than on the therapy delivered.

The remaining two-thirds of patients (16) had no metastases identified in 2 to 11 nodes harvested. Because it has not been the recommendation of our institution for patients who have node-negative colon cancer to receive chemotherapy, these patients would be at risk of being undertreated.[8]

To address the concerns raised by this finding, the pathology department has developed a colon cancer protocol that requires repeating the search for lymph nodes after placing the mesenteric tissue in an alcohol, formaldehyde, and glacial acetic acid mixture (Dissect Aid) for all cases having fewer than 12 nodes identified. This solution produces a pale white appearance in nodes, which facilitates their identification. If this further preparation still yields fewer than 12 nodes, representative sections of the mesenteric adipose tissue are submitted for review. In cases in which the final pathology report still shows fewer than 12 nodes, the pathologist contacts the surgeon to recommend a medical oncology referral to discuss whether the patient should receive adjuvant chemotherapy.

Since the publication of the COST study in 2004, laparoscopic colon resections for cancer have increased greatly.[9] Initial examination of our data by the Colorectal Disease Site Group identified a disturbing trend regarding node harvest when open colon resections were compared with laparoscopic resections. Of those node negative cases in which fewer than 12 nodes were evaluated, 56% were performed laparoscopically. For this reason, demonstration of proficiency with 15 nonmalignant laparoscopic colectomies was proposed by the Site Group as a prerequisite for the use of the laparoscopic approach for malignant tumors by surgeons at our institution.[10–12] Because the sample size of the CP3R was small, we decided to examine records and pathology reports for all colon cancer cases in 2008 and 2009 to have a direct comparison between open and laparoscopic resections (see **Tables 3–5**) before finalizing this proposal. The results of this comparison suggested that the laparoscopically resected specimens were smaller than those of open resections for right hemicolectomies, but that this discrepancy did not seem to affect the node harvest. For the left-sided resections, there were fewer lymph nodes removed for the laparoscopic group (13.8 vs 17), but this difference was not statistically significant. There were significantly more nodes removed when the colectomy was performed for right-sided tumors than for left-sided lesions (see **Table 4**), and the percentage of patients having 12 or more nodes removed was significantly higher for lesions on the right side, no matter which surgical technique was used. On average, both groups still exceeded the 12 nodes required by the NQF standard, with 74.5% of left colectomies and 88.2% of right colectomies meeting this standard. The explanation for the differences between right-sided and left-sided procedures is not clear but it may simply be caused by nodes being less abundant on the left side. It has been our impression that the mesentery to the descending colon and splenic flexure is often thin, with sparse nodal content. Another explanation could be that deep pelvic nodes may be difficult to retrieve by either surgical approach. There does not seem to be a difference that can be attributed to the operative approach selected by the surgeon. As a result, our criteria for credentialing surgeons for laparoscopic colectomy have not changed.

SUMMARY

Review of the NQF measures for colon and rectal cancer provided to COC-accredited programs by the NCDB can provide clues to deficiencies in care that can be addressed by multidisciplinary actions. We have used these measures to assess care at a community-based teaching hospital to try to improve the uniformity and quality of care delivered by a diverse surgical faculty. In rectal cancer, the NCDB data for our institution showed 100% compliance with the use of radiation for the conditions indicated (American Joint Committee on Cancer [AJCC] T4N0M0 or stage III rectal cancers), but surprisingly small numbers of eligible patients. Review of the accessioned patients showed that, in many cases, patients were ineligible because the recorded stage was too early to justify the inclusion of radiation in the treatment protocol, partly because we had insufficient pretreatment staging, and we have introduced enhanced pretreatment staging measures to address this problem.

Review of our node harvest in colon cancer has led to enhanced procedures for pathologic specimen preparation to maximize chances of retrieving the required 12 nodes. When these added measures still do not result in identification of 12 nodes, communication of this information from the pathologist to the surgeon is now required to allow for timely referral of the patient to receive chemotherapy even when the nodes do not show metastatic spread. A direct comparison of node harvest by laparoscopic technique versus open technique in nearly 200 colon cases has raised the issue of potentially inadequate node retrieval in left-sided colectomies, but this difference does not seem related to the surgical techniques used and may be caused by there being fewer nodes to harvest on the left side.

REFERENCES

1. Reproduced with permission from the NCCN Complete library of NCCN clinical practice guidelines in oncology. National Comprehensive Cancer Network; 2009. Available at: http://www.nccn.org. Accessed (Month and Day, Year). To view the most recent and complete version of the guideline, go online to www.nccn.org. Accessed October 1, 2010.
2. Wallengren NO, Holtas S, Andren-Sandberg A, et al. Rectal carcinoma: double-contrast MR imaging for preoperative staging. Radiology 2000;215:108–14.
3. Urban M, Rosen HR, Hobling N, et al. MR imaging for the preoperative planning of sphincter-saving surgery for tumors of the lower third of the rectum; use of intravenous and endorectal contrast materials. Radiology 2000;214:503–8.
4. Lahaye MJ, Engelen SM, Nelemans PJ, et al. Imaging for predicting the risk factors-the circumferential resection margin and nodal disease-of local recurrence in rectal cancer: a meta-analysis. Semin Ultrasound CT MR 2005;26:259–68.
5. Brown G, Kirkham A, Williams GT, et al. High-resolution MRI of the anatomy important in total mesorectal excision of the rectum. Am J Roentgenol 2004; 182:431–9.
6. Blomqvist L, Holm T, Rubio C, et al. Rectal tumours–MR imaging with endorectal and/or phased-array coils, and histopathological staging on giant sections. A comparative study. Acta Radiol 1997;38:437–44.
7. MERCURY Study Group. Diagnostic accuracy of preoperative magnetic resonance imaging in predicting curative resection of rectal cancer: prospective observational study. Br Med J 2006;33:779–82.
8. Swanson RS, Compton CC, Stewart AK, et al. The prognosis of T3N0 colon cancer is dependent on the number of lymph nodes examined. Ann Surg Oncol 2003;10:65–71.
9. Clinical Outcomes of Surgical Therapy Study Group. A comparison of laparoscopically assisted and open colectomy for colon cancer. N Engl J Med 2004; 350:2050–9.

10. Tekkis PP, Senagore AJ, Delaney CP, et al. Evaluation of the learning curve in laparoscopic colorectal surgery: comparison of right-sided and left-sided resections. Ann Surg 2005;242:83–91.

11. Dincler S, Koller MT, Steurer J. Multidimensional analysis of learning curves in laparoscopic sigmoid resection: eight-year results. Dis Colon Rectum 2003;46: 1371–9.

12. Schlachta CM, Mamazza J, Seshadri PA, et al. Defining a learning curve for laparoscopic colorectal resections. Dis Colon Rectum 2001;44:217–22.

Index

Note: Page numbers of article titles are in **boldface** type.

A

Ablation. *See* Hepatic tumor ablation.
Accreditation, National Accreditation Program for Breast Centers, **581–586**
    for community-based cancer center programs, 418
Adoptive cellular therapy, of cancer, 548–549
Adoptive immunotherapy, for cancer, 541–544
Allogeneic vaccines, in cancer immunotherapy, 539–540
Allovectin-7, in cancer immunotherapy, 538–539
American College of Surgeons Commission on Cancer (CoC), analysis of performance
    among cancer programs in different categories of CoC accreditation, 556–567
        demographics, 557–559
        five-year survival data, 564–567
        mission of CoC, 556–557
        National Quality Forum measures, 559–562
        surgical treatment administered, 562–564
    role in building a community-based cancer center program, **417–425**
        Accreditation Program, 418
        cancer center categories, 419, 423–424
        cancer center *vs.* cancer program, 418
        cancer program categories, 419, 420–422
American College of Surgeons Oncology Group, and the community surgeon, **439–445**
American Society of Breast Surgeons, Mastery of Breast Surgery Program, 570–573
        benefits of participation, 572–573
        expanded program, 572
        pilot program, 571
Antibody-mediated immunotherapy, for cancer, 541–544

B

Benchmark, for cancer care, breast conservation therapy *vs.* mastectomy in
    community-based cancer centers, **427–437**
Bevacizumab, in cancer immunotherapy, 546–547
Boards. *See* Tumor boards.
Breast cancer, care in community-based cancer centers, **427–437, 467–485, 555–580,**
    581–586
        breast conservation therapy *vs.* mastectomy, **427–437**
        challenges, opportunities, and outcomes of, **555–580**
            American Society of Breast Surgeons and Mastery of Breast Surgery Program,
                570–573
            analysis of performance among different types of cancer programs, 556–567
            job description for community breast surgeon, 567–568
            measuring outcomes in, 573–576

Surg Oncol Clin N Am 20 (2011) 597–603
doi:10.1016/S1055-3207(11)00025-1
1055-3207/11/$ – see front matter © 2011 Elsevier Inc. All rights reserved.

surgonc.theclinics.com

Moving?

Make sure your subscription moves with you!

To notify us of your new address, find your **Clinics Account Number** (located on your mailing label above your name), and contact customer service at:

Email: journalscustomerservice-usa@elsevier.com

800-654-2452 (subscribers in the U.S. & Canada)
314-447-8871 (subscribers outside of the U.S. & Canada)

Fax number: 314-447-8029

Elsevier Health Sciences Division
Subscription Customer Service
3251 Riverport Lane
Maryland Heights, MO 63043

*To ensure uninterrupted delivery of your subscription, please notify us at least 4 weeks in advance of move.

Printed and bound by CPI Group (UK) Ltd, Croydon, CR0 4YY

03/10/2024

01040448-0017